EMPOWERED MEDICINE

HARNESSING THE INFINITE LAWS OF THE UNIVERSE FOR OPTIMIZED HEALTH

TRIP GOOLSBY, MD & LENAE GOOLSBY, JD

BALBOA
PRESS
A DIVISION OF HAY HOUSE

Scripture taken from the Holy Bible, NEW INTERNATIONAL VERSION®. Copyright © 1973, 1978, 1984, 2011 by Biblica, Inc. All rights reserved worldwide. Used by permission. NEW INTERNATIONAL VERSION® and NIV® are registered trademarks of Biblica, Inc. Use of either trademark for the offering of goods or services requires the prior written consent of Biblica US, Inc.

Balboa Press books may be ordered through booksellers or by contacting:

Balboa Press
A Division of Hay House
1663 Liberty Drive
Bloomington, IN 47403
www.balboapress.com
1 (877) 407-4847

Print information available on the last page.

ISBN: 978-1-5043-8536-7 (sc)
ISBN: 978-1-5043-8537-4 (e)

Balboa Press rev. date: 09/28/2017

To the seekers of a better way to motivate and heal themselves of illness and disease. To the visionaries who are willing and able to see and achieve optimized health and longevity. To those brave patient-partners whom we have met along our journey who are willing to share the stories of their own personal journeys toward healing their health and their lives.

I do not believe—indeed I deem it a comic blunder to believe—that the exercise of reason is sufficient to explain our condition and, where necessary, remedy it, but I do believe the exercise of reason is at all times necessary.

—Peter Medawar,
Nobel Prize winner and author of *Advice to a Young Scientist.*

CONTENTS

PREFACE

At the turn of the twentieth century, William James, godson of Ralph Waldo Emerson, stated, "The greatest revolution of our generation is the discovery that human beings, by changing the inner attitudes of their minds, can change the outer aspect of their lives." In light of this and similar thoughts found in various writings throughout history, I wonder why it has taken us so long to incorporate mind-body approaches into the practice of traditional medicine. Use of prescription drugs dominates our current approach to treating illness, despite abundant evidence that behavioral modification may work just as well, and without causing unwanted side effects.

I believe part of the reason for this is that physicians are trained to prescribe treatments based on peer-reviewed studies that demonstrate positive outcomes with the use of certain medications. Although researchers and participants in the studies are presumed to have no impact on the outcome of the studies, this presumption is in error, and this error is known to have existed since the early twentieth century.

When we see positive results with the use of a placebo or inexplicable positive outcomes with health-related affirmations, we must admit there is a mind-over-health connection that is manifesting itself in the form of unexplainable outcomes.

Is it possible that the inexplicable positive outcomes attributed to a placebo are related to our error of interpretation of the data, an error of interpretation of the true effect? Could not the positive outcomes result from the participants' anticipated outcomes—the "mind-body" effect? I believe our health and well-being are actually being forced to respond to our beliefs and desires by virtue of what we think, or expect our health to be, the result of a mechanism of our own volition. This is also, all biological behavior being equal, the explanation for many of the significant differences in outcomes for people, despite having similar disease stages in cancer. I have observed these same differential responses in both my oncology and integrative medicine patients with chronic disease processes over the years.

Is it simply a lack of knowledge of our ability to contribute to the "happy end result" that is slowing down our ability to move into a quantum medical outcome? I would say, yes. I would also say that the existence of an understandable systematic approach, one that provides us with a simplified means of motivated and empowered behavior adjustment, will significantly improve our outcomes. As Gregg Braden, author of *The Spontaneous Healing of Belief*, stated, "The act of us simply looking at our world—projecting the feelings and beliefs that we have as we focus our awareness on the particles that the universe is made of—changes those particles as we are looking."

Before moving on, I would like to tell you more about myself. In the fall of 1975, I started to pursue my dream of becoming a physician. Unlike most, I began by acquiring French as a second language. I did this because my family expatriated to Belgium in the service of an international petroleum corporation when I started college two years earlier; the advantages of being considered a Belgian national for the purposes of education benefits could not be ignored. After successfully completing my studies at the Universite Libre de Bruxelles, I completed my internship in internal medicine and residency training at the University of Health Sciences/Chicago Medical School, and a fellowship in oncology and hematology at Roswell Park Memorial Institute and the State University of New York at Buffalo.

Along the way, through my professional endeavors, I was blessed with meeting the love of my life, LeNae. We met through a mutual acquaintance at a restaurant in Murfreesboro, Tennessee, in early 1998. The meeting was quite brief, and I recall thinking that a young woman of such incredible beauty could not possibly be attracted by a nerdy geek such as myself. My inner child helped me escape from the scene after brief social pleasantries, in which all abilities to speak the English language coherently left the scene more rapidly than my motorcycle, which followed shortly thereafter. My social awkwardness notwithstanding, LeNae salvaged the encounter when she called my practice the following day. Uncharacteristically so, the gatekeepers transferred her call back to me.

She didn't even give me a chance to ask her out. I suspect she preferred not to distract me from my professional obligations and preempted what would have surely been another embarrassing moment for me by asking me if I might like to go to dinner sometime to continue the scintillating conversation we had engaged in the day before. She reminds me, to my continued embarrassment, that my response was an astonished guffaw, followed by a really fast, "Yes, I'd love to!"

Five years of dating later, and an equally clumsy proposal to LeNae produced marriage and a number of marvelous perspectives and outcomes in my life. These miracles are the origin of a multitude of awakenings and enlightenments that contributed to the origin of this book and the methods I use to inspire, empower, and enhance the acquisition of significantly improved health outcomes for my patients.

The first enlightenment, and quite frankly one I thought was not going to happen during my life for numerous reasons, was the conception of our son, Henry IV; not that the biology and the chemistry weren't there, by any means. I'd maintained the limiting belief that being a good father and the demands that I imposed upon myself to provide best outcomes for my patients were incompatible. I stopped believing this on the eve of my fiftieth birthday, and Hayden Granger (aka Huckleberry) followed less than four years later.

At that time, my interest in health optimization reached its peak. I started investigating peer-reviewed new age therapeutic methods that could minimize the ravages of time on our physical bodies and perpetuate a dynamic health span.

This study led me to acquire additional certifications, which I incorporated into my oncology practice. The successes experienced by my oncology patients were quite impressive and gratifying, so I began expanding my integrative medicine practice, using the techniques and data I had gathered. This was quite fortunate, as discord was brewing in the wings of my medical partnership. Putting my family above my affiliated nursing staff and colleagues caused conflict and provided a catalyst for change. This priority shift and awakened purpose also provided insight into the transformational and motivational components in this book.

My transformation and understanding came more from the personal effort and struggle that was the result of my lifetime *change*. I became endowed with the perspective necessary to see a body of motivational and transformational literature that has been the source of success for thousands—possibly millions—of individuals all over the world, and for millennia.

Although these transformational success methods were not previously specifically used in the setting of disease management, it occurred to me that the major chronic illnesses (those most effectively reversed by an optimized integrative approach, such as diabetes, cardiovascular disease, hypertension, depression, anxiety, among others) were a ripe field for an empowerment approach that could motivate and assist in the transformation of lifestyle attitudes and habits that were the result of misinformation and/or limiting beliefs about our health.

In my mind's eye, I envision a type of "motivational medicine," a "transformational mindfulness," to enhance and empower those who are discouraged or defeated by conventional medicine. Or, quite frankly, for those who are so accustomed to the current mode of mass production reactive healthcare delivery that they don't even know that they are, themselves, the source of creation of a better health. I see how this approach may serve to enhance treatments and increase the likelihood of an empowered mind-body response.

Almost as though I had spoken the words aloud, LeNae enrolled in a number of intuitive-empowerment training programs. I naturally became curious and began reading a number of the authors whose titles are familiar to those seeking answers in the domain of personal development and intuitive empowerment. These references led to my attending lectures and reading other authors. I gained a historical, philosophical, and religious review that reached back into pre-antiquity and encompassed a number of spiritual, religious, and metaphysical viewpoints. These methods dovetail quite easily with those of therapeutic imaging and biological feedback, as well as the other contemplative and mindfulness modalities. They likewise are the source of this empowered approach that, in my hands, and at this writing, anecdotally is generating virtually unheard levels of compliance and enthusiasm for personal health and well-being transformation.

By traveling on this avenue, I collided with a number of the new thought, personal success, and mindfulness authors (Allen, Shinn, Hill, Proctor, Emerson, Byrne, Dyer, Chopra, Dagher, Braden, Massaro, Canfield, Ziglar, and others). After LeNae took an online study course on the work of Raymond Holliwell, offered by Bob Proctor and Mary Morrissey, LeNae and I decided to write this book.

How can we best learn about and embrace the changes necessary to succeed in improving or eliminating detrimental habits? What can we reasonably expect to achieve when implementing a motivational behavior modification program? I see the use of the universal laws as a means of mindful, transformational motivation bring about and improve adherence to change. The principles of these laws have been used in diverse cultures over the millennia to captivate and motivate humanity. Some name three universal laws. Others name twelve, and some, as many as twenty. These laws include the law of attraction, which states that our thoughts, feelings, words, and actions produce energies that attract like energies. Negative energies attract negative energies, and positive energies attract positives energies. In this book, I have identified twelve universal laws that relate to achieving optimal health, one for each chapter.

The universal laws have a substantial foundation in all of our cultures, religions, and backgrounds, dating far back into antiquity. In Christianity, for example, there is the principle of sowing and reaping—people reap what they sow, so it's wise to sow positive things. These motivational and lifeward principles are espoused by psychological, neuropsychological, and motivational leaders of our times. They are used to help those who are aware of the need, in many domains, to make change. Change is necessary to rid ourselves of bad habits we have acquired that cause us to have many of the chronic illnesses that plague our society.

Using the universal laws with my patients as a pathway toward understanding how we create our health (good or bad) has been an epiphany for both patient and physician (me) alike. Their ease of use by patient, counselor, and physician can enhance personal resolve, accountability, and discipline to acquire new behaviors and achieve improved outcomes in virtually anyone willing to participate. I believe, however, that using the empowered, compassionate guidance of a "practitioner-coach" is by far the most effective in achieving the optimum outcome. The "practitioner-coach" scenario facilitates the creation of intention, which is the sum of belief + motivation + resolve. This brings about a greater potential for the quantum observer effect: the act of observation causes change to that which is observed. This applies to both the practitioner, who believes change and improvement is possible, and to the patient, who desires, believes, and intends to achieve change.

I progressively incorporated this empowered motivational training alongside the medical and lifestyle methods of my integrative practice. Our 4-Pillar Approaco care includes transformational mind-body medicine, nutrition, physical fitness and exercise, and hormonal and metabolic optimization. This gives way to a significant improvement in quality of life while easily transitioning the majority of my patients off most of their prescription medications for chronic diseases, such as diabetes and hypertension.

Ultimately, this integrative medical practice gave birth to what is now Infinite Health Integrative Medical Center in both New Orleans and Lake Charles, Louisiana. We are avidly developing as we help patients to become empowered creators of their own health, improving their attitudes, outlook, and lives while eliminating the need for toxic pharmaceutical medication by lifestyle measures, bioidentical hormonal and metabolic optimization, as well as motivational, transformational contemplative practices.

Using empowered motivation eases anxiety and reduces the failure and noncompliance in anyone who desires better health. Our program at Infinite Health employs universal laws applied to the patient's specific medical situation, and does so in a logical sequence. Using this same approach permits us to address patient-specific habitual weakness in the areas of compliance and resolve that often leads to failure in efforts that are unassisted by similar approaches. The simple addition of daily mindfulness and contemplative imaging techniques makes these changes easier to accomplish. Although there is certainly a single institution and investigator bias included in the examples given here, I am confident that the individual who desires real and effective change in life for better health may be effectively empowered and transformed by the use of this methodology. My wife, LeNae, and I have written this book to help people understand this approach so they can obtain empowerment to achieve healing of illness along with the long-lasting quality of life we all deserve.

—Trip Goolsby, MD

INTRODUCTION

The greatest revolution of our generation is the discovery that human beings, by changing the inner attitudes of their minds, can change the outer aspects of their lives.

This quote, attributed to both William James and Albert Schweitzer, highlights the force contained in an empowered mind-body approach applied to any facet of our lives, not just our health. It also seemingly shares the frustration of a practical wisdom that the author wishes to impart to those who would benefit greatly from this empowering perspective. If we are spiritual/energetic beings living a physical experience, and one of our purposes is to advance or learn during our time in our physical embodiment, then in order to accomplish new learning, we should be provided with an option for information acquisition and advancement.

Many of the challenges and efforts necessary for us to achieve success from the initial implementation of any therapeutic plan require powerful motivation and dedication on the part of our partners involved in the healing endeavor. The more complicated the case, and numerous the conditions, the greater the energy and motivation required to achieve success. The awareness and mindfulness provided by the following chapters will empower each person who engages in the exercises to accomplish his or her desired health goals.

In the advancement of knowledge is sheltered the need of knowledge without perception of need. So many of us pass through the gate of learning by stumbling or falling. The broken hip from osteoporosis is the result of hormonal deficiencies associated with advancing age. The onset of diabetes is the end of the path of the hormonal imbalance of aging, along with detrimental nutritional habits, and, in most cases, long-standing obesity. These examples stem from the unknown need for knowledge that is not perceived until our youthful reserve is largely consumed and the symptoms of a disease process are upon us. It is then, in the best of reactive fashion, that we say, "Oh, it happened all at once." Doctor Google becomes our best friend, and we just as suddenly have a store of knowledge that resembles our physician's. To our great misfortune, however, we have adopted a multitude of lifestyle customs that are of questionable benefit at best.

In *Empowered Medicine*, we have summarized a template of empowerment, a pathway successfully used by many of our patients in achieving virtually any health care goal upon which they have focused. It is our intention here to facilitate a clear understanding of the concepts that many of our patients have questioned along their own journey. In my practice, Infinite Health Integrative Medicine Center, with two offices, one in New Orleans and the other in Lake Charles, Louisiana, much of our time is spent on interpreting the practical meaning of universal laws in the context of individual challenges. In this book, we will explain these laws so that you may gain a more practical ability to apply them to your own medical problems and practice them for optimized health. More significant than physical exams and the review of laboratory and imaging abnormalities, adaptation to the concepts of personal health creativity has been the true turning point for the majority of my patients. That is to say, in the long term, more health optimization success is obtained when clear pictures of the rules of engagement are generated and a clear image of the desired outcome is created.

The concepts of the universal laws provided herein are often poorly understood and/or poorly incorporated into the daily thought processes, behaviors, and habits of most people. Because of this, we experience challenges in our ability to create our preferred lifetime experiences, not only as they relate to lifestyle desires, but also in the optimization of health and wellness. Generating a clarified meaning and concept in the mind is therefore one of the most empowering exercises we can accomplish by using these laws we engage in an empowered transformational mindfulness that gives perspective, alleviates stress, and raise our vibrational energy helping us acquire the successful health image we desire, therein making us the creators of our health.

Dr. Deepak Chopra expressed it well when he related, "Everything that exists in the physical world, is the result of the unmanifest transforming itself into the manifest … anything and everything that we can perceive through our senses—is the transformation of the unmanifest, unknown and invisible into the manifest, known, and visible." This correlates well with the fact that we are continually transforming our bodies by virtue of the environment we create inside ourselves through our nutrition, our exposures, and the internal responses we generate to the interactions we experience in the world around us on a continuing basis. These internal responses create processes that either help us and heal us, or make us ill. They are also the source of empowerment and enable us to achieve whatever outcome we desire for our health.

What is the reasoning behind the treatment and lifestyle changes that many of us must implement to succeed at health optimization?

There are two main issues: genetic blueprints and one's functional reserve. We inherit a set of genetic blueprints from our parents that are the templates for our lives, health, and well-being.

This is our DNA (deoxyribonucleic acid). If we respect the blueprint and avoid creating an abusive interpretation of it, we stay happy longer. If we disrespect it on an ongoing basis, we reap what we sow.

There is a reason we don't feel as well as we were accustomed to feeling earlier in our lives. It is not, however, simply because we are older. Certainly, time has its sacred role in the evolution of our sense of well-being, but only to the degree that the choices we make create the outcomes of our desires, passive or active. Ralph Waldo Emerson, related in his discourse on compensation, "A perfect equity adjusts its balance in all parts of life. '*Oi chusoi Dios aei enpiptousi!*' The dice of God are always loaded." And, in the case of the human being, the balance of the outcome is such that we may effectively improve our health and longevity by sowing the right seeds. As Mr. Emerson so astutely noted, in this way we know we will always be compensated for the way we live our lives and the choices we make (or the ones we avoid making).

Biologically, we are also aware that our organs allow us the largest of an impressive "functional reserve." This reserve is permissive. Even when we eliminate up to eighty percent or more of an organ's function, we may do so without endangering our ability to survive. We may, in fact, continue to thrive, improve, and perform on a relatively high level with this level of organ function. Eliminate one or two more percent from this marginal function, and there it is, a symptom, malaise, illness, disease, and, most importantly, a loss of the sense of invulnerability that accompanies our youth.

We try to bring back the vigor of our youth by increasing the duration of our exercise, changing what we eat, and, more often now, by taking multiple supplements and nutraceuticals (nutrients with claimed or proven results that do not require a prescription). The question that is foremost on our minds here is, "What will enhance our waning stamina and our sense of well-being and take us back to the 'glory days'?" The answer is usually provided by our integrative physician, first in the form of corrective lifestyle changes and then with medication, if necessary.

The accompanying question that must always be answered in kind is, "What are *we* willing to *change* to get back there?" It is in answering this question that the insight and motivation provided by this book will be the most useful.

In becoming more mindful of how we achieve the discipline and motivation, we provide ourselves fuel for the motor of change. Using this fuel has assisted not only those who wish to recover from significant disease but also those who, with foresight, are instead focusing more intensely on how to slow down or prevent loss.

We now have the knowledge that subtle changes occurring in multiple different laboratory parameters are associated with a silent but clinically meaningful decline in our longevity and quality of life as we reel in the years.

Most of the healthier parameters replicate our more youthful years; for example, maintaining certain hormone levels in the upper twenty percentile of our lifetime values yields decreased risk of heart attack and stroke. This same optimization yields a robust and substantial improvement in our sense of well-being and also sustains a biologically youthful vascular infrastructure.

The information that manages our reserve is received from our parents and is encoded in our DNA. DNA is associated with numerous proteins and enzymes that form twenty-three pairs of chromosomes. The Human Genome Project, completed in 2001, found approximately twenty-three thousand genes. This is referred to as our genome. These genes, by the process of transcription, lead to the formation of an as-of-yet-unknown total number of proteins. (The sum total of proteins transcribed from our DNA is called the proteome.) Estimates are that there are somewhere from 150,000 to two million proteins that may be formed and incorporated into a human body.

How is this possible? That is, how is it possible that twenty-three thousand genes can produce that many different proteins? It is possible because our genome is available for interpretation and expression by a complex system of reactions that has been called *epigenetics*. This is where I would like to introduce EVE: epigenetic variability effector.

EVE is the personalized concept of an intelligent sum of molecular biological activities that may improve, leave unchanged, or compromise the function of the cell into which information is provided. Based on the influences that each of the cells in our bodies is subjected to, their individual epigenetic infrastructure interprets and guides the subsequent biomolecular events that yield positive or negative DNA expression and interpretation; for example, protein products to be transcribed from the genome. That is to say, EVE will be either happy, angry, or unmoved by the statements made and provided by the outside world (food, ingested or inhaled toxins, radiation energy from the sun, and other stimuli) or by the inside world (metabolic and hormonal changes due to ever-present responses of our minds and bodies to the interactions with the world around us and our thoughts and imaginations). These byproducts will then go on to influence the positive or negative outcome of the cell, it's survival, and, ultimately, the survival of the individual.

Some of these changes are short lived—one or two cell cycles, depending on the exposure or the local environment. Some, however, may be imprinted for the lifetime of the individual and one or two generations thereafter.

The information that produces epigenetic modulations may be from inside the body or outside the body. Ultimately, it is this input of information that exacts the beneficial, neutral, or adversarial impact on all of the cells of the body.

Information from outside the body is easy enough for most of us to conceptualize. Many nutritional, pharmaceutical, physical, infectious, and toxic agents may play roles in the manipulation of our epigenetic manifestations. In actuality, the field of nutritional epigenomics is just beginning to yield fruit through studies involving the elemental content of food substrates. These elements are then assessed to appreciate the effects they have on DNA expression, and ultimately how they lead to pathways that may improve individual well-being. Suffice it to say, we may soon potentially be able to choose our meals to modulate whatever part of our genome we wish.

The influence of information from inside the body derives primarily from our hormonal and autonomic nervous system and the influence their actions may have on the organs that maintain life. This system, described further in chapter two, is of primordial importance and will be the focus of the exercises in this text. The sum of these epigenetic modulations will eventually yield an environment that either consumes, ignores, or improves the reserve of our different organ systems.

Reading and using the exercises provided in this book will usher in enhanced abilities to focus on desired outcomes and the means to attain them. It will be a means by which we may all be empowered to not only achieve the health we desire but to activate our imaginations and beliefs to manifest the environment and trappings of that successful health image. It is an important affirmative, mindful, complementary step in the direction of self-realized health, healing, and well-being, harnessing empowered awareness to acquire the long-lasting quality of life and the healing of illness we all deserve.

CHAPTER 1

The Infinite Law of Success in Health

If we did all the things we are capable of doing,
we would literally astound ourselves.

—Thomas A. Edison

Fran (all patient names in this book are fictional) was seventy-eight years old when we first met. Actually, she didn't meet me until a number of days after her admission to the hospital. Her habitually limited quality of life had recently been compromised by a state of septic shock, a severe bacterial infection that causes the heart to fail and the blood pressure to drop severely, causing the body's internal environment to become incompatible with life. She had been surviving, up until about two to three days earlier, with multiple medical issues, including severe obesity; adult onset diabetes complicated by nerve, kidney, and eye damage; vascular disease; and coronary artery disease. She underwent a triple bypass operation four or five years previously, and her last echocardiogram indicated congestive heart failure. Additionally, she had chronic obstructive pulmonary disease (COPD), degenerative arthritis of her lower back and knees, gout, and rheumatoid arthritis.

She was transferred to me from an outlying community when her compromised kidney abilities and heart failure caused accumulation of the chemotherapy in her body, leading to bone marrow failure with subsequent elimination of all the white blood cells (the ones that protect us from infection) and platelets (small cells that plug the holes when we start bleeding) in her body. Amazingly, my colleagues and I were able to salvage her marrow function while providing medications to stimulate the fabrication of new white blood cells and transfusions of red blood cells and platelets, all the while covering her with industrial doses of antibiotics and antifungal medications that were eventually necessary.

She was able to greet me for the first time only about eight days after her admission, when she no longer required the use of the ventilator or blood pressure support. Thereafter, she recovered slowly, in the hospital at first, and then at home, for the following month to six weeks.

When I first saw her as an outpatient, she was remarkably frail and wheelchair bound, mobilizing only with the aid of her three daughters, who lived near her. She was, however, quite lucid and expressed the sincere desire to recover as much of her former physical function as possible, if not to improve upon it. She had gardened avidly when she was healthier and imagined that a return to that—or something better—would be a desirable lifestyle accomplishment that she had not appreciated in some two to three years.

We worked collaboratively for the following ten months, using a multifaceted, optimized nutrition, exercise, and an endocrine approach that was the source of some concern for family members. The nutritional approach was a low-carbohydrate one, which resulted in a resolution of the need for insulin supplementation and all but one of three oral medications for blood sugar control. Because Fran was postmenopausal, I prescribed female bioidentical hormone replacement therapy and also optimized her thyroid hormones and adrenal substrates. Two of her three daughters were opposed to any exercise, believing that Fran's multiple conditions precluded anything but the most limited physical activity. Gardening, they felt, was without a doubt out of the question as was the use of any aerobic exercise equipment. Concerned about pain from her arthritic afflictions and the daughters' contrary beliefs that Fran would surely have a heart attack, they argued against any such interventions. They also argued against any additional hormones fearing, in their misinformation, that she would have complications from their usage.

I insisted, however, that acquiring any improvement in her overall condition would necessitate progressive incremental efforts along with the nutritional, nutraceutical, and hormonal manipulations.

I thought two of Fran's three daughters would lynch me before the end of that day when I discussed the initial plan and the rationale. Had it not been for the intervention of the eldest daughter, who took away their rope, I might not have survived to write this vignette! Fran's image of success was to be better than she was prior to her hospitalization, and I was determined to facilitate that image, as long as it didn't cost me my life.

Fran was all in. Her vision of success was clear. She provided the effort and forgave the two younger daughters' limited beliefs in her abilities. She worked to her maximum capacity at all times; her image of success was ambulation and independence in the home setting, walking to the daughters' houses, which were in reasonably close proximity, and planting and managing the garden of her dreams again without assistance.

A year after Fran's hospitalization, she *walked* into my office with the aid of only a cane. She was frequently walking to her daughters' houses nearby, and she was out gardening as she saw fit, to the amazement—and appreciation—of the younger daughters. Given the nature of her accomplishments, I was also curious to evaluate her cardiopulmonary recovery, as she was no longer short of breath when she walked. I suggested we obtain a follow-up echocardiogram to assess her left ventricular ejection fraction (heart function efficiency testing). It had improved! New tests showed an amazing 38 percent, although the previous test in the hospital had shown 18 percent! She experienced many other functional improvements that accompanied a significantly improved quality of life, and she continued to improve even more thereafter. A number of other medications related to blood pressure and arthritis were also reduced and/or discontinued during this same period.

Fran remains, for me, one of the most poignant examples of how much we may truly accomplish in the face of devastating and debilitating chronic disease processes when using an approach that focuses on the desires we have to achieve a specific vision of health success. This is a simple case, but I think it illustrates what an optimized integrative approach can achieve.

It is clear that we are all created capable of having the health we desire in that we live, for the most part, for years and years without the slightest hint of encumbrance. This period of grace is more or less dependent on the genetic gifts of our parents to us (our genomes) combined with the abuse to which we subject our particular genome. Finally, when we have exhausted most or all the reserve we were gifted with at birth, we develop symptoms and signs of disease. But this is not the end. Even at the point where disease (dis-ease) becomes apparent, we may recover a significant degree, if not all, of our health by successfully committing to a guided program of recovery. Many of us want to do just that when we receive the wake-up call. This turning point emerges and allows us to change direction and obtain different outcomes. For those of us who understand this nature of our underlying reserve, or who are fortunate enough to work with a practitioner who is prepared to assist in optimizing the reserve in lieu of simply giving another pill, we become the master of our future health outcome to the degree our reserve permits. How do we know what that reserve is? This will be clarified in the forthcoming chapters.

We are born with incredible resilience and flexibility in recovering from injury and insults of many types. The plasticity of the different organ systems and their ability to recover is inborn and always ready to respond, adapt, and help us recover from even the most catastrophic events. Many individuals in our Infinite Health programs are aware of this and use this recovery potential to great advantage. The Infinite Health programs are individually created for health optimization based on the individual medical issues and information of each patient. Our personalized mind-body approach is also tailored to the specific challenges of each patient and woven into the foundation of the eleven laws coaching format, which is adapted dynamically based on the individual and his or her responses and situational challenges throughout the course of care.

Each of us has the potential for seemingly endless improvement from any aspect of our lives. This ability is a natural process that is defined and contained in our respective genetic makeup. Understanding the nature of this self-empowering gift gives us the robust ability to succeed at any convalescent recovery (or any other endeavor) we choose. I allude here to the simple effect that we see in athletic circles about record-setting performances. Regardless of the level attained by one athlete, there is always—and will always be—an improved performance eventually.

Some of you may be thinking that your ability to recover or improve is beyond your physical capacity. I can assure you, you will be reflecting, as did Mr. Edison in the opening statement, "If we did all the things we are capable of doing, we would literally astound ourselves." But, in order to achieve this, you must follow your earnest desires and use the universal laws to embolden your behavior and connect yourself to the source of all that becomes real and tangible in our existence.

If nature—the universe—is ignorant of failure, it is because she recognizes that all the natural universal laws are always working together to enhance our health. Furthermore, it is when we are simultaneously in harmony with these natural—or universal—laws that we become an indistinguishable force of creation. With that empowerment, we are never limited in our abilities to recover, improve, and develop our health: *No matter where we are when we begin, we will yield a successful outcome!* Recent research into how our internal and external environments manipulate our bodies' genetic makeup confirms this statement. Epigenetic changes based on the environment that bathes our cells can recreate our bodies over time—to our benefit or to our detriment. It's our choice!

When we understand and collectively implement these universal laws, the probability of success is significantly greater. The reason for this is that learning, adapting, and adhering to these laws gives us the knowledge and ability to work in harmony with the forces of universal good and creation. We'll accomplish the results by conforming to a new behavioral foundation that empowers us to grow and advance by harmonious cooperation with the laws of nature and the universe.

Most of us aspire to improved health and a more durable, high-quality life. Not unlike the successful business executive or professional, we are better served and we have fewer chances of failure if we have *guidelines by which a successful outcome might be obtained*. Using these laws will help us to establish a correct understanding of the principles upon which successful achievement might be founded. And those achievements will lead to the healthier, longer lifestyle—what I like to call "health span"—that we desire.

So, what is success? Defined as the favorable or prosperous termination or completion of attempts or endeavors or the accomplishment of one's goals, success is clearly dependent upon the beliefs of the individual contemplating the question. It depends on perspective and originating viewpoint, as well as whether or not the individual believes his or her efforts related to the endeavor are complete. Understanding that we have an unlimited availability of resources and that we can support this with a limitless desire to complete whatever effort we have undertaken, we need to admit that we can achieve whatever goals we determine for ourselves. What does success look like for you?

> *What is success? To laugh often and much; To win the respect of intelligent people and the affection of children; To earn the appreciation of honest critics and endure the betrayal of false friends; To appreciate beauty; To find the best in others; To leave the world a bit better, whether by a healthy child, a garden patch or a redeemed social condition; To know even one life has breathed easier because you have lived; This is to have succeeded.*
>
> —Ralph Waldo Emerson

This understanding, ultimately, should come to us as the result of our own logic, cognitive, and intuitive abilities. What I frequently see, however, is that we often sell ourselves short from a lack of understanding of what we are capable of, or from the imposed beliefs of others that we have assumed to be true. When applied to our lives, however, these assumed limiting beliefs are invariably only hypothetical, unsubstantiated, and ultimately untrue. When, on the other hand, we affirm, by desire and heartfelt intuition, our ability to succeed, we also invariably set and subsequently attain our goals!

The indispensable first step to getting the things you want out of life is this: Decide what you want.
—Ben Stein

Yes, we can have any success in health we desire by providing the effort necessary to arrive at the goal. Desire is like the gas that powers the engine of advance so that we continue to move forward toward the determined goal. That desire must power the action of attainment by virtue of generating the initiative to achieve new foundations of personal preparedness and ability. We are, all of us, capable of developing our hidden talents, intellect, intuition, and our hidden and unknown strengths in the pursuit of the health-related goals we desire to achieve to be successful. Vision and intention are the keys that will provide access to the energy of desire. They are the universal resources that subsidize success. And that success is valid for any health-related desire we so choose.

> *No person can succeed who is not imbued with the desire to advance … The*
> *desire to advance implies the power to advance … The fact that you desire to*
> *succeed is evidence that you have the power to succeed; otherwise, you would not*
> *have been urged to aspire success-ward.*
> —Raymond Holliwell, author of *Working with the Law:*
> *11 Truth Principles for Successful Living*

In terms of advancement, continued progress in the direction of our goals is the yardstick necessary to define success or impending failure. By definition, when we have terminated all effort that defines forward progress, then, and only then, have we failed. It is only in expending energy in the direction of the established goal, or in accepting the challenge of a temporary failure as a means to a better outcome, that we are able to advance. This means that, while en route to the health we wish to achieve, we may need to learn new things. For example, learning how to get onto the Internet and research things that help to achieve our happy end results is a good thing! We may need to establish a new plan for advance after a setback, seek advice from an esteemed advisor or a member of our health care team, and so forth.

Setting small goals that draw us ever closer to the final one is sometimes the most critical of approaches that should be considered in our advance toward success. This enables us to celebrate intermediate successes as we assimilate the elephant in small bites. Many who are dealing with longstanding chronic health problems will benefit from this approach. Setting small goals also allows for smaller setbacks if there is a minor failure; that is, the "indigestion" (frustration) will be more tolerable along the way.

> *If you want to be happy, set a goal that commands your thoughts,*
> *liberates your energy, and inspires your hopes.*
> —Andrew Carnegie

The law of success is defined by this forward unstoppable momentum, not unlike the laws of nature. Whatever we imagine as our success in terms of our health is what we are capable of achieving (you will see this again in the law of supply).

We should never be fearful of the greatest imagined outcome that we can intuitively create, as this is what we will always be able to actualize going forward. The reason for this is that we have within ourselves the ability to learn, create, and improve upon ourselves to achieve virtually any physical, emotional, and mental demeanor that we can imagine. The empowered desire of our heart is given to us only because we are capable of achieving it. We are additionally always connected to the resources necessary to build the physical products of our imaginations and, therefore, our health.

If we imagine intuitively (in our hearts and mind) that we are capable of achieving a goal for our health, we can, and then some. Proverbs 4:23 reads, "Guard your heart above all else, for everything you do flows from it."

This would seem to imply that, if we establish our goal and plan of action from the sincerity of the heart, and our thoughts and subsequent actions remain in keeping with our integrity of purpose, success is assured.

That being said, we might be upset along our path by obstacles that appear, particularly if we are not abiding by the principles that help us keep our thoughts centered on our goals.

Fear of success—or failure—is a detrimental obstacle, and we must not allow it to enter into our stream of consciousness. And why should it? When Source has provided us with the image of success, there is no obstacle that can withstand this assisting force.

In the following poem by Guillaume Appolinaire, I often see the interaction I have with many of my less-well-initiated patients, as well as those individuals who are scarred as a result of multiple setbacks and/or "failures." It is interesting how well the laws support and empower these individuals from their perches on the edge of another attempt.

Take a Leap of Faith and Fly!
"Come to the edge," he said.
We can't, we're afraid," they responded.
"Come to the edge," he said.
And so they came.
And he pushed them.
And they flew.

There is an abundance of good-health potential even in the severely ill. This is a known quantity that has been demonstrated time and time again. Consider the multitude of clinical vignettes centered around individuals paralyzed following strokes who subsequently recover to live virtually normal or normal lives. Think also of athletes condemned never to compete again who miraculously compete—and win! Or even think of the story of Fran. The first months after her discharge, I must admit that my own belief faltered at times. The simple fact that we have such a reservoir enables and then empowers the desire to achieve; it fuels the inexhaustible fire of reserve to succeed, so much so that we need only to think, speak, and act as if we have it already for it to be so (see the law of supply).

Trip Goolsby, MD & LeNae Goolsby, JD

> *Believe and act as if it were impossible to fail.*
> —Charles F. Kettering

I am amazed at the variability displayed in the outward demeanor of different people who are approaching their individual health challenges, and then following the outcomes they subsequently achieve. These final outcomes that I have observed are clearly attached to individual patients' thoughts, attitudes, and beliefs, specifically as they relate to their successful health image.

The most important of the attitudes necessary for success is the attitude of "I can!" Most often, this thought process determines outcomes of a positive nature by instilling the desire and initiative necessary to overcome major and minor obstacles, along the path to the desired goal. The momentum generated by "I can!" delivers on the promise of inspiration and empowered creativity. Affirming, "I can!" helps to produce the ideas that can resolve the roadblocks that often slow the progress along the pathway to success.

> *Nothing can stop the man with the right mental attitude from achieving his goal;*
> *nothing on earth can help the man with the wrong mental attitude.*
> —Thomas Jefferson

Those who have a lifestyle that gave them a chronic disease process that is killing them do not have to remain anchored to that lifestyle until their ultimate demise is achieved. We do not need to think we can't change, or that we cannot be successful because we have "always done it this way, or that way." We are all amazing infinite beings who are gifted with the capacity to assess challenges and change our erroneous behavior at will. All of our brains contain that ability; we need only call upon the two little words that deliver the power to drive desire and the momentum of change for the acquisition of the health we want. And those two words are, *I can!* We are, thus, all of us, capable of success in our health, whatever health we may choose!

Thinking
by Walter D. Wintle

If you think you are beaten, you are,
If you think you dare not, you don't,
If you'd like to win, but think you can't
It's almost a cinch, you won't.

If you think you'll lose, you're lost,
For out in the world we find,
Success begins with a fellow's will
It's all in the state of mind.

If you think you're outclassed, you are,
You've got to think high to rise.
You've got to be sure of yourself before
You can ever win a prize.

Life's battles don't always go
To the stronger or faster man,
But soon or late the man who wins
Is the man WHO THINKS HE CAN!

We screen patient-partner applicants at Infinite Health to determine their level of desire and attitude. Interestingly, many of the patients who initially believe they cannot succeed, when coached on the implication of the negative attitude, are able to shift into a can-do attitude and succeed over time. This depends, of course, on the level of desire for positive outcome. We gauge desire and motivation on a simple one-to-ten subjective scale, as is attitude. Additionally we like to inform patients that the phrase "I can't!" must be eliminated from their vocabulary during their time at Infinite Health, and particularly during the timing of their training!

The simple use of the phrase, "I can!" generates an empowering positive attitude that can be felt simply in the utterance of the words. In fact, it is an exercise we do when discussing this chapter at the beginning of the mind-body program. That is, when we engage our affirmative ability to accomplish anything related to our health, our creativity and determination are enhanced to formulate a path toward the successful completion of the imagined goal. In that affirmation we create the image of the victorious conqueror who creates and summons all of the necessary resources and relations to thrive.

Your Empowered Medicine Cabinet

The Lotus of Life Personal Self-Assessment

It is often helpful to have a visual reference for where we may need to shift our focus and energies with respect to the various aspects and demands of our lives and the toll they may be taking on our health

This Lotus of Life personal self-assessment is designed to do just that. By taking fifteen to twenty minutes to go through the following aspects of your life, you will gain a better picture—perhaps even a larger perspective—of where you are rocking things, where you may be coasting, and finally where the balls may be dropping.

A perfect life is going to look like a perfectly circular lotus flower. If, after completing this personal self-assessment, your lotus is perfect, let's meet for lunch 'cause, beautiful, you need to be coaching me. If, however, there are some dips and divots, no worries at all. This does not mean you are failing at a single thing; it is merely informational feedback designed to allow you to choose where you may want to redirect your energy.

For each of the following categories below, rate yourself on a scale of one to ten. One is very poor, five is neutral, and ten is awesome and amazing.

Once you have rated yourself (do it honestly, because this is for you—and you know, to your own self be true), divide each category by ten. For example, if under the "Family" category you have a 70, divide that by ten to get 7.0.

Then, take the 7.0 and plot it out on the lotus petal for "Family." Once all categories are complete and plotted on the lotus, connect the dots. That's it! Easy breezy!

Spiritual

Belief in a divine creator_____

Faith _____

Intuitive_____

Sense of freedom to speak authentically _____

Inner peace _____

Compassion _____

Sense of personal power _____

Sense of personal creativity_____

Sense of feeling belongingness_____

Other_____

Total: _____ Divided by 10 = _____

Self-love

Daily fun activity_____

Fitness/exercise _____

Spend time with friends_____

Practice random acts of giving _____

Open to receiving_____

Spend time in meditation/reading _____

Practice prayer/gratitude _____

Spend time in personal development _____

Make nourishing choices_____

Other_____

Total: _____ Divided by 10 = _____

Family

Strong family relationships_____

Feel respect _____

Feel accepted_____

Feel heard _____

Feel supported _____

Quality time together _____

Vacations _____

Constructively resolve differences _____

Affectionate_____

Other_____

Total: _____ Divided by 10 = _____

Mental

Positive attitude_____

Logical/critical thinker _____

Creative/emotional _____

Strong formal education _____

Continuing education endeavors _____

Reader _____

Puzzles/games/brain exercises _____

Artistic/creative endeavors _____

Self-image_____

Other_____

Total: _____ Divided by 10 = _____

Physical health

Happy with physical appearance_____

Strong energy and endurance _____

Positive results from regular checkups _____

Involved in an integrative health program _____

Taking zero prescription medications _____

Engage in regular fitness activity _____

Healthy BMI _____

Good genes _____

Positive self-talk_____

Other_____

Total: _____ Divided by 10 = _____

Career

Love what you do _____

Exceed expectations _____

Positive colleague relationships_____
Feel like you fit with the team _____
Receive constructive feedback _____
Continuing training/education _____
Take leadership opportunities _____
Feel supported/valued _____
Aligned with company goals/vision/mission_____
Other_____

Total: _____ Divided by 10 = _____

Financial

Happy with income _____
Multiple revenue streams _____
Have clear financial goals and plan_____
Have and stay within budget _____
Have financial investments _____
Have savings account(s) _____
Have life/health insurances _____
Zero credit debt _____
Pay obligations on time_____
Other_____

Total: _____ Divided by 10 = _____

Great job! Now take your results and plot them out on the lotus to get the full picture of where your opportunities for improvement are!

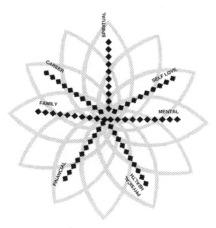

CHAPTER 2

The Infinite Law of Thinking in Health

All that we are is the result of what we have thought; it is founded on our thoughts; it is made up of our thoughts.

—Buddha

Gregg is an interesting patient. He reflects on occasion about how his multiple chronic medical problems have nothing to do with his ability to prevent them. His mother raised him as the "sickly sibling," chanting frequently to him, "Oh, Greg, you've always been a sickly child, and you always will be." Defending his multiple maladies he states, "That's how I've always been, and I always will be. It's not my fault!"

He missed a follow-up appointment, having been admitted to the hospital for a bout of acute pancreatitis. The pancreas became severely inflamed and painful causing nausea, vomiting, severe abdominal pain, and jaundice in his case. Sometimes, pancreatitis causes more severe problems and even death. His reflections were similar when he returned three weeks later to see me. "I had nothing to do with it," he affirmed, although he underwent surgery to remove his gallbladder for gallstones, and a blockage of his common bile duct (the channel leading from the liver to the small bowel through the pancreas). The blockage was at the origin of the episode of acute pancreatitis. He was, by his declaration, completely unaware of the role he had in the creation of his disease process.

Point in fact, Gregg had a number of health conditions and lifestyle activities that predisposed him to gallstones and precipitated the subsequent attack of acute pancreatitis. Those conditions were largely associated with his morbid obesity, adult onset diabetes, as well as a diet that contained excessive amounts of carbohydrates (dietary sugars) and virtually no fiber. He also had hyperlipidemia, a condition associated with multiple different fat types being too concentrated in the blood, and hypercholesterolemia, too much cholesterol in the bloodstream, which had yet to be properly corrected despite his taking cholesterol-lowering medications (another risk factor for gallstones). Other medical conditions plaguing Gregg's sense of well-being were hypogonadism (undiagnosed and untreated inadequate sexual hormone concentrations), hypertension, suboptimally treated hypothyroidism (low thyroid output), and severe degenerative arthritis.

Gregg was completely unaware of the multiple roles he had played in creating his gallbladder stones. This ignorance regrettably made him no less guilty of being the proximal cause of creation of the stones that resulted in his hospitalization and subsequent surgery. His thought processes and decisions had created the damaging lifestyle that led to the poor nutritional and activity patterns in his life. These finally resulted in the compromise of his gallbladder and liver function responsible for the formation of the stones. Acceptance of his mother's statement was simply a passive decision to defer causality resulting from uncaring ignorance of fact.

> *Sin, sickness, sorrow and affliction do not, in reality, belong to the universal order, are not inherent in the nature of things, but are the direct outcome of our ignorance of the right relations of things.*
> —James Allen, author of *From Poverty to Power* (1901)

The universal law of thinking tells us that the customary thoughts we have create the foundations for the outcomes of our lives. Thought has always been recognized, in a spiritual sense, as the causality and creator of effect.

> *Spiritual truth is always at work, beyond what the eye can see … Our interaction with the spiritual world is governed by our thoughts. When we know this truth and consciously align our thoughts with it —sometimes even despite how we feel—we activate its spiritual power. We transform our mortal circumstances by bringing our thoughts about them into alignment with a world that lies beyond.*
> —Marianne Williamson,
> author of *The Law of Divine Compensation*

Every thought creates something by virtue of its energy. On a rudimentary and practical note, to clarify the fact that thought produces something, it is known that new thoughts create new neurological connections, and ultimately the repetition of thoughts may create new complex nervous pathways (synapses) in the brain. That means a collection of neurons (brain cells) is being created as we take new actions and establish new healthy habits. On the physical plane, thoughts travel with the speed of electrons (light). The energy of thought is then interpreted by the formula $E=mc^2$. Understandably, the mass of an electron is not truly substantial. It is, however, the cumulative effect of thought that produces significant mass and establishes the existence of new substance.

It is of utmost importance that we realize thinking and thought are the primary drivers of our health. It is the thinking that we do that is responsible for our subsequent actions and habits. These actions and habits are beneficial, empowering, and support the health and lifestyles that we possess. Or, they may be detrimental beyond repair. (Here I'm thinking of smoking and other self-abusive activities that we acquire over the course of our lifetimes).

If we read these lines carefully, we become energized and enamored with the subtle notion these printed words carry. That notion is that our inborn possession of extraordinary abilities can create whatever health we choose from whatever health we have. I appreciate this same thing clinically in my biased patient population. Biased here refers to the patients in my practice who are more creative and successful because of the empowering assistance of my support team and myself. This is the same health-bound creativity that abides in these laws and originates from sometimes near-catastrophic clinical situations, both physical and emotional.

We are the creators of our lives! We are the art and the artists! We create this art in many ways and by many means, but it all starts from the first constructive thought of improvement. The effects of our creative abilities are being confirmed and catalogued virtually daily by medical science and technology. The medical science that confirms the effect of our thoughts on our health assaults both physician and nonphysician alike on the same daily basis. If we go to Google Scholar and query "stress with disease" we receive 3,400,000 scholarly articles that contain this relevant term! (Google Scholar can be found at https://scholar.google.com/). Cancer, heart disease, stroke, diabetes, hypertension—there are thousands of related clinical trials, and all of them are related in some shape, form, or fashion to the thoughts we have.

What are the important elements that enable and empower us to pursue improved outcomes? Which ones help and which are of little, zero, or nefarious benefit? Clearly, with the amount of available scientific information alone, the assistance of mentors and well-versed clinicians is necessary for all who wish to avoid the consequences of being ignorant of what optimized health thoughts consists of. We must remain alert for the significant thoughts, actions, habits, and character traits that will usher in benefits.

Thinking and Its Effects

There is a marvelous inner world that exists within man, and the revelation of such a world enables a man to do, to attain, and to achieve anything he desires within the bounds or limits of Nature.
—Raymond Holliwell, author of *Working with the Law:*
11 Truth Principles for Successful Living

So what is a thought, or idea? What is thinking? A thought is defined at Dictionary.com as: "any conception existing in the mind as the result of mental understanding, awareness, or activity" or "any mental representational image of some object or action."

Ideas can also be abstract concepts that present as mental images: the mental images of things not currently seen or sensed by the sense organs. It is not by coincidence, then, that the premise attributed to William James (and Albert Schweitzer), which came about some five thousand years following the conclusion drawn by Hermes Trismegistus (3000–5000 BC), are virtually identical with that of Trismegistus: "The greatest revolution of our generation is the discovery that human beings, by changing the inner attitudes of their minds, can change the outer aspects of their lives."

Thinking is the act of producing thoughts. These thoughts are ideas, or collections of ideas, themselves the result of thinking. Although this seems to be a bit redundant, it really is insightful. Thinking produces a number of results, both immediate and long term:

1) **Actions:** This is the simplest immediate result of thought. We do not move our hands or feet without the presence of a preceding thought, no matter how fleeting and unperceived.

2) **Emotions:** More complex in their nature and appearance, emotions involve the instinctual state of mind. The combination of your experiences and the feelings associated with those experiences define your thought response. This thought response is subsequently communicated to additional areas of the brain by means of holographic patterning, which produces three-dimensional images in the brain. The areas involved in the hologram, which may be activated repeatedly in some instances, are based on our past thoughts and current beliefs. They are positive (and health generating) or negative (and health detrimental).

3) **Beliefs:** Simplistically, these are personal truths birthed out of repeated thoughts.

Belief is the state of mind in which a person thinks something to be the case, with or without there being empirical evidence to prove that something is the case with factual certainty.

—Wikipedia

Beliefs may be beneficial or detrimental, but they do not necessarily represent truth. This last point is important for us to remember. Beliefs guide our thoughts and our conscious activities. They lead to actions in order to produce demonstrable effects, thereby reinforcing or compromising their existence. They are the stuff that impresses our minds with the motivation to accomplish any goal or image that we may produce or desire in the mind's eye. They are also the source of emotional responses that may improve or compromise our health, as we will see later. Importantly, any desire to change our health or outcome from any intervention whatsoever, by necessity, must be accompanied by an appropriate belief that is subsidized by the correct thought processes that will engage, reinforce, and empower the change. For example, if we want to lose weight, we must tell ourselves that it is possible, that we know what we must do, and that we are willing to do it. We cannot go around telling ourselves, or others, that it's impossible for us to lose weight, or complain about how hard it is to lose weight, while simultaneously expecting to lose weight.

The principle to the approach we use at Infinite Health is to orient and empower a focus on the desired health outcome that is believed attainable. We assist our patient-partners in creating an image that, because we help resolve limiting, disempowering beliefs, is significantly better than the patient originally created. This empowering approach is based on actual outcomes available to the individuals that they may be completely unaware of during their initial consultations. Changing our thoughts from the health we have to a focus that helps obtain our desired outcome requires modifying our behavior and energetic focus. Although our initial goals and beliefs may be somewhat tarnished (limited) by our past experiences—and this is the case with most all of us—in the context of our unknown abilities, our bodies are capable of far more than we may initially believe. Our vision and sense of empowerment grows rapidly with the success we progressively obtain, rest assured.

Many in the new thought arena allude to the disbelief of personal ability to achieve whatever desired goal as a "limiting belief" because it is just that. Limiting beliefs are the beliefs that limit our potential best outcome, disempowering us to the point of failure. How do we really know whether we can or we cannot? In many situations, some of us reject the possibilities for improvement out of hand. I am no longer able to count the number of cases I have witnessed of patients saying, "I can't," only to achieve the positive outcome. This often happens within a few months of the statement. A "poor" mechanic once said, "Whether you believe you can or you can't, you're right." That was Henry Ford. There are any number of methods to overcome these annoying obstacles to our best health.

The perfect example here is John, a sixty-plus pack-year smoker (two packs of cigarettes per day for over thirty years). John was quite excited to improve upon his existing health. He presented with mild to moderate COPD (chronic obstructive lung disease) and a number of other chronic health issues. He stated that his motivation level to feel better was an eight out of ten. When told he would be required to cease all tobacco consumption to succeed in obtaining his desired optimized health image, he could only say, "I can't do that, Doc." I thought he would walk out of the office mad at the staff and me, but we managed to reach an agreement after his lung testing came back. He understood his levels of activity were being sorely restricted by his limited lung reserve, and I reminded him of how he was making EVE mad and what she was going to continue to do. He quit smoking within four months without the use of any medication. This exemplifies perfectly what altering a belief that would otherwise compromise an optimized outcome can do.

Continuing our list, now, thinking also produces:

4) **Attitudes:** These result from the interaction of our past thoughts and experiences in the present to create a favorable, or unfavorable, disposition toward a person, place, or thing. This is our judgmental ego posturing and is reflected by how we behave.
5) **Habits:** Repeated actions become habits (for better or for worse), and the combination of our multiple habits and beliefs define our character.
6) **Character:** The combination of our multiple habits and beliefs.
7) **Destiny:** As we apply our character—and therefore the sum of our habits and beliefs— to the events and challenges of our lifetime, we determine the outcome, consequences, or destiny of our lives.

This sequence of events holds true as well for the character of our health and well-being. For this reason, applying our thoughts, related to the universal laws, defines our health destiny. This effect illustrates our ability to determine the outcome of our health by the quantum nature of existence. That is to say, you have and are in control of this effect at all times. In this sense, in the quantum-based sense of reality in which we live, we are the artist and the art of our lives. We are not simply the Newtonian victims of happenstance, observers in the void watching the goings-on of reality. We are effective instruments that impose thoughts, beliefs, and character, as it were, on ourselves, and our environment (bodies), the surrounding that is molded by our intent.

Thoughts, then, are substantial forces; they are created by us to do our bidding. One hundred years ago, the basic sciences, through the work of brilliant physicists such as Max Planck, Albert Einstein, Niels Bohr, Werner Heisenberg, and Erwin Schrödinger, determined that thought and belief directly influenced the outcomes of scientific experiments (quantum physics). Current research into the effects of mind on health will probably disclose the "placebo effect" as the effect of our minds (thoughts, attitudes, and beliefs) on our health. What this means is that what you think about in terms of your health, you bring about. The biological changes brought about by new constructive thought processes about your health will provide for healthier outcomes.

What this also means is that the thoughts and beliefs of your physician, health care practitioners, or any other person who may provide you with health-related information and care have the potential to impact your ability to arrive at your desired outcome.

Your thoughts are a materially creative power in that they will produce new synapses (connections between nerves), new neurons (nerve cells), new epigenetic modifications of your genes (controlling factors that make your DNA express itself in different, more constructive ways). So, ultimately, the improved modifications of your body will follow. All of these changes are themselves representative of behavioral changes that will modify your physical body and being, and will then significantly improve your health and quality of life.

> *Imagination is everything. It is the preview of life's coming attractions.*
> —Albert Einstein

You are the result of all of your thoughts and beliefs up to this moment. This statement is so profound that it would truly take hours or chapters to detail. Suffice it to say, every action we take for our health requires a preceding thought. Repetitive thoughts about our health that are founded in similar informational background lead to beliefs about our health. Depending on the source and veracity of the information, the belief will be either beneficial or detrimental in nature. Repetitive actions of a similar nature lead to health-related habits. These are also good or bad, depending on the information and its related source. Habits and beliefs lead to the formation of a particular mental disposition (character) toward good or poor health which, when applied to all lifetime situations, leads to a certain fitness destiny.

It is in this setting that Professor Einstein's quote is so important. Our imagination for our ultimate health and well-being is simply the preview of what we may obtain. So, we must use our created image to our best advantage.

One of our biggest challenges is to take the knowledge base we have of our current health problems, along with the conscious and subconscious images we have developed of them, and establish a new image and thought pattern both consciously and subconsciously. While we are unaware of negative subconscious images, we can still replace them with positive ones by rebuilding our conscious thought patterns. The most important contributor to our health, or our ability to improve our health consistently, resides in the customary thoughts and beliefs that we hold, as well as the customary thoughts and beliefs that our treating healthcare providers hold for us. The relative medical parameters (diagnostic, prognostic, therapeutic, and so forth) of our ongoing medical issues will also be strongly colored by the information we are given by our health care providers.

Should our physician be of a nihilistic bent (having an attitude that life has little or no meaning, extreme negativity, pessimism, or cynicism), manifest by little or no concern or compassion for our condition, we will be better served to choose one who will work in the direction of our desired health image. The reason some physicians have this type of attitude is that they are unable to stay abreast of the massive amount of information being produced in the different domains, and more so, they are unable to correctly interpret the data, particularly given the caveat of quantum perspectives that is not being accounted for. The academic literature is also replete with discussions of practitioner nihilism in many branches of medicine (neurological disease, cancer, vascular and heart disease, and so forth). It is for this reason that, when we derive our image of improved health, the practitioner who advises us should be aware of the relative data, or be willing to review it, and be capable of empowering our image to achieve the best outcome with patience and compassion. Start somewhere and improve the image as you improve. How many times does the artist refine the outline or dabble with the color before the final image becomes acceptable to him or her?

In the event that the physician has embraced an integrative practice, the coloring may be somewhat more favorable than it would be in the setting of a traditional reactive medical practitioner. The information and participation by reactive practitioners is, in most cases, quite limited given the restricted amount of time devoted to the development of a comprehensive diagnostic and therapeutic plan with the patient. After all, how can a comprehensive a plan be developed when the national average visit time for an internist/primary care practitioner in the United States is only seven minutes?

As we follow the guidelines of an empowered success-based universal laws program, the process retrains our thoughts and perspectives to recognize spontaneous behaviors that do not serve our best health. We also begin to seek out the beneficial behaviors that drive our well-being, mind, body, and soul, to levels that we left behind in our youth (or maybe never had).

Most behavioral modification programs require 21 to 260 days to accomplish the task of a change in habits. More people trend toward the 180–250 day mark, and require significant "support" to make it happen.

Even though the events and biological nature of thinking are actively being dissected on a macroscopic, microscopic, and molecular biologic level, we are yet in the early stages of understanding these elements. Pharmacologic development and many clinical trials will be necessary before we amass the robust data required to produce therapeutic drug manipulations that would be truly fruitful in the practical setting. And, really, why do we need to give up the power of our bodies and minds to the corporate accounts of the pharmaceutical industry? Why, indeed, when technology such as functional MRI and other imaging studies are delineating more clearly different areas of the brain that are active during different emotions and responses to different stressors?

Further, studies that dissect the molecular and epigenetic changes (DNA expression and activity modifiers) that an individual may experience during different types of thought are also bearing fruit. All these are interesting but far from a practical pharmaceutical product, whose implementation would garner substantial and meaningful benefit in the domain of sustainable behavioral modification. Realistically again, that "pill" may not necessarily replace the natural ability we have, ourselves, to modify our own health-related behavior, particularly if a simple, practical, and effective system is available. I hesitate to imagine the necessary length of the television ad that would be able to intimate at even the minority of the side effects and toxicities that such a product would have! Lastly, pharmaceutical agents are unlikely to be capable of modifying our beliefs such as they are. This is a crucial area that remains the domain of subconscious suggestion and repetition that, when successful, replaces the nefarious behavior with a new constructive one.

> *What you are, so is your world … It matters little what is without, for it is all a reflection of your own consciousness. It matters everything what you are within, for everything without will be mirrored and colored accordingly.*
>
> —James Allen

When we review and reconsider this, and the earlier quote from James Allen, we understand that he is telling us we can harness the power of our thought to keep us from illness and help us avoid and/or heal sickness using the power of mind. Thus, by replacing ignorance with knowledge and then applying that knowledge to our best effect, we participate in the creation of our destiny. This could be the "quantum" interpretation and effect of Mr. Allen's thought.

Imaginative Mental Chatter (the Monkey Brain) and the Stress Response

Our brains and minds are the amazing tools that serve us and evolve with us (and for us) throughout our lives. We are capable of teaching them, and therefore helping them (and us, as a result) evolve, as long as we draw breath. This means we are blessed with the ability to create whatever person, with whatever abilities, we so choose. The key to this ability is to learn how to find and remove our limiting thoughts and beliefs. These are the thoughts and beliefs that are erroneous or founded in harmfully damaging information. We must replace them with the affirmative, empowering ideas that create the infrastructure most apt to provide us with optimum health.

The way we integrate events and information about our health into our minds guides us more than anything else does to the creation of this foundation of empowering wellness. This groundwork takes its shape progressively over the course of our lives by virtue of our lifetime experiences. Primarily, and for the most part, we acquire good or bad information as children, and the quality (beneficial or not) of this information is dependent upon how—and from whom—we received it. It is subsequently reinforced, by trial and error, over the course of our lives.

Ideally, as children, we would be best served if we were all fed an informational diet of well-formulated healthy thoughts based upon robust, critically peer-reviewed health information. This information would be reinforced by new reviews of pertinent information at the time we need to make any new health-related decision that would affect our immediate or long-term well-being. Of course, not all of us had well-versed, objective, caring, and enlightened physicians as parents from whom we could glean, or who would provide us with reliable, robust health-related information when we were children. Even if we did, they probably weren't home much, and the information would be sorely outdated by now.

The point is, action does not take place until a related idea or thought is germinated. These ideas will have been critically conditioned by our health- and wellness-related beliefs (our past, if you will). The natural law of thinking is conditioned by belief in such a way that our thoughts and ideas are subjugated by them, and therefore, so are our health-related decisions and actions.

Most of our modern-day thinking is a complicated mixture of spontaneous inner dialogue. I refer to this as chatter, or the monkey brain. This is the incessant babble that is the construct of our "reality" meshed with egocentric creativity, and that, in most cases, is hypothetical hyperbole. This ego-based activity is the fertile compost of our experiences. Like it or not, the monkey brain creates a morass of mischievous meanderings that can derail constructive thought and belief, potentially guiding us into an imbroglio of unhealthy behavior.

*I have had a lot of worries in my life,
most of which never happened.*

—Mark Twain

Know this: you are actually in complete control of your monkey brain, and your health is not subject to its frenetic fiction unless you focus on and anticipate the outcome it presents to you.

Let's look at the effects of the monkey brain when it presents us with a stressful scenario. As Mr. Twain so eloquently clarified for us, the vast majority of our stressful exposures in life come from our own imaginations. It is as though the monkey brain is determined to play scenario after scenario of a hypothetical, emotion-wrenching soap opera and violence-ridden reality television program for our amusement. The unfortunate part about this is that we are the stars of the soap opera fantasies, and the human brain possesses a limited response profile in the setting of stress. The stress response for any *imagined* incident is identical to that of a *real* incident, so you get the same physiological response whether the sabertooth tiger is actually right there in front of you, or only there on the "screen" of your mind.

What Happens to Our Bodies When We Respond to Stress?

As we think—and we are almost always thinking of something because of the incessant chatter—our brains provide us (our minds at any rate) with a synthesis of the information by virtue of an integration of what our senses perceive. The mind, using filtering based on its lifetime experiences, integrates the information presented to it. Mind, however, is also quite creative, as you may realize. It has the ability to create or imagine situations that are then perceived as real. So our minds are not very critical or discerning; in fact, they pretty much respond the same way to input received by the senses as they do to input created by our imaginations.

Any situational disturbance of the equilibrium that exists between an organism and its environment is termed "stress." Stressors are the information gathered at the level of the cortex of the brain from the sensory organs, or they are created by our imaginations. They are subsequently assessed as threatening or not, and forwarded to the amygdala, the brain's center for emotional input. This emotional message is then passed on to the hypothalamus with subsequent activation of the autonomic and parasympathetic nervous systems, which are the nervous pathways that emit signals to bring about the responses of body organs, for example, to change the blood pressure and/or increase the heart rate and rate of breathing.

The hypothalamus also sends messages to the pituitary gland by releasing multiple hormones designed to release more hormones. The anterior pituitary relays further hormonal messages to the body with multiple responses taking place at the level of the targeted organs. In so doing, they effectuate and perpetuate the cortical interpretation of the stress.

Because these responses are created on an ongoing basis, the hypothalamus integrates and qualifies the stress as being acute (short term) or chronic (of long duration). The stress response then elicits the following hormone releases from the hypothalamus: corticotrophin releasing hormone (CRH), which stimulates the release of adrenocorticotropic hormone (ACTH) from the pituitary gland); antidiuretic hormone (ADH), which is also known as vasopressin (ADH acts on the kidney to promote water retention); gonadotropin releasing hormone (GnRH), which stimulates production and release of luteinizing hormone (LH) and follicle stimulating hormone (FSH), both of which act on the ovary or testicles; and lastly, thyrotropin releasing hormone (TRH).These hormones then elicit release of adrenocorticotropic hormone (ACTH), growth hormone (GH), thyroid stimulating hormone (TSH), prolactin, 8-lipotropin, 3-endorphin, follicle-stimulating hormone (FSH) and luteinizing hormone (LH), all of which act on their respective glands to create the optimum environment in the body that will help sustain survival when the saber tooth tiger attacks.

In the acute adversarial stress reaction, cortisol is one of the main hormones released by the adrenal glands under the effect of ACTH. Cortisol's task is to regulate blood pressure and the glucose (sugar) levels in the bloodstream in order to keep the body alert and vigilant. It blocks the activity of insulin, keeping blood sugars levels high for immediate use as an energy source. Chronic stress and the cortisol response related to prolonged adrenal stimulation are associated with aggravation of diabetes, hypertension, and severe immune compromise that may accelerate the advance of cancer.

Next in the order of significant hormones that are released during a stress response are the catecholamine derivatives. These are predominantly represented by epinephrine (adrenaline), and norepinephrine. The activities of these hormones bring about an increase of blood flow to the heart, brain, skeletal muscles, as well as increasing the diameter of the airways for better breathing. They also help retain sodium by the kidney, which increases fluid volume in the blood vessels for improved blood flow into the vital organs. Catecholamine activity tends to diminish blood flow to those organs less in demand during fight or flight. (After all, do we truly need to worry about the kidneys or how nice our skin looks when the grizzly is taking his first bite?) Both of these hormones also block the action of insulin and increase the amount of sugar available as an energy source. (Sweet-and-sour sauce for the tiger?) Thyroid hormones, insulin, and the gonadotropins FSH and LH levels are decreased in adversarial stress responses, while those of growth hormone and prolactin are increased.

Interestingly, although it is well known that chronic stress can induce abnormalities of the menstrual cycle including complete impairment of reproductive function, the decrease of these two hormones (FSH and LH) in men likewise result in significant reductions of serum testosterone levels under the similar circumstances. (Who needs libido while dodging the claws?) And while the level of growth hormone is significantly increased during acute stress reactions, chronic stress causes significant decreases in growth hormone production and secretion. This is important, particularly with respect to our body's ability to repair itself.

In 2007, Cohen, Janicki-Deverts, and Miller published an article on psychological stress and disease in the *Journal of the American Medical Association* (JAMA). In the setting of chronic stress, they reported the effects of chronic elevations of many of the stress-related hormones, as well as the inappropriate decreases in activity of other hormones. Chronic stress can lead to the further compromise and worsening of many chronic diseases such as chronic fatigue, hypertension, obesity, diabetes, anxiety, irritability, and depression. It can also compromise metabolic and reproductive functions as well as the immune system.

Insofar as clinical outcomes are concerned, we are more often focused on negative outcomes. When we are able to focus on positive outcomes, then we eliminate the repetitive activation of the stress response. We then enhance the body's natural healing tenancy and encourage the immune system to act in concert with therapy.

Providing the ability to achieve a proactive, positive mindset necessitates different levels of intervention. The simple administration of medication is not always successful in achieving this effect. I have observed this over years in the setting of cancer chemotherapy administration. Some patients are not always capable of altering their mindset or thought patterns into a more constructive or positive view. These patients are then, regardless of pharmaceutical assistance, destined to drift toward the more adverse outcomes. Not infrequently, an adverse prognoses from misinformed family members or a nihilistic or uninformed physician has significant detrimental impact on survival and quality of life, despite positive response to therapy.

> *Let a man realize his life, in its totality, proceeds from his mind, and that mind is a combination of habits which he can, by patient effort, modify to any extent, and over which he can thus gain complete ascendancy and control, and he has at once obtained possession of the key that shall open the door of his complete emancipation.*
> —James Allen, author of *Out from the Heart*

It is in the James Allen sense that the more beneficial effects of the law of thinking should be taken. The law of thinking is defined as the universal principle that defines thought (thinking, imaging, imagining, and so forth) as the invariable or consistent (in any setting conceivable) and repetitive process, determining the lifetime conditions (destiny) of woman and man. It is by corollary that our dominant thoughts and their consequences determine our health as well.

You have been inspired to read *Empowered Medicine* for a specific reason, and that reason is precisely why you will be able to achieve any outcome of success in health that you desire. Do you think to yourself, "There is a better 'me' in there somewhere, and I would really like to be that 'unique empowered me' that has a higher quality of life, a better energy level, a better physique, a happier sex life, the ability to be more active and thriving as I mature"? We think, and rightly so, that we possess a unique ability to change. With that thought, we activate the means by which we will achieve the desired outcome. We obtain our goals, not only by changing our thoughts about our health, but also by controlling them in a way that will bring about the metamorphosis we desire—eliminating the monkey brain, calamity, chatter thinking.

Empowering ourselves along the path to the image of our optimized health requires a usable framework—or guidelines if you will—for how we should pursue a great outcome, or avoid a bad one for that matter. That is where Empowered Medicine comes in.

> *It is the nature of mind to create its own conditions, and to choose the states in which it shall dwell. It also has the power to alter any condition and to abandon any state, and this it is continually doing as it gathers knowledge of state after state, by repeated choice and exhaustive experience.*
> —James Allen, author of *Out from the Heart*

In Luke 17:21, Jesus says, "The kingdom of God is within you" (KJV). This notion of a state of heavenly existence may be interpreted as being related to the nature of our inner consciousness, the conscious or subconscious thoughts that we maintain on an ongoing basis. It is related to our personal state of mindfulness. The more peaceful, constructive, healthy, and orderly our consciousness, the more perfected—heavenly, conscious, aware, mindful—life we will experience. These are the same empowered thoughts that lead to our optimum health. These types of guiding, mindful, enlightened, productive thoughts then usher us into the achievement of all things. The guidance of the verse from Luke is reinforced by Matthew 6:33:, "Seek ye first the Kingdom (the thoughts and attitudes of mindfulness and enlightenment) of Heaven (consciousness) and all things will be added." This insightful guidance tells us that heaven is attained by an orderly, disciplined state of mind, the focal point of which is on those desirable qualities of the "kingdom," or empowered, enlightened thought, as opposed to the mundane "needs" of daily living. For our health, the extrapolation is the same. Our mindful, enlightened, informed thoughts and ideas take us to our desired destination of well-being.

The mandate here that guides our thinking is that we need to organize and focus on the universal laws; only then may all of the attributes of excellent health be acquired. Being in tune with these qualities empowers and guides us to universal gifts, perfect healing, and fitness. That said, if our minds were to guide us to maintain an organized, disciplined, and proactive vision of our positive, happy end game (excellence in health), we would more easily achieve it. Refer again to the James Allen quote above.

If we are easily distracted, emotional, short tempered, prideful, envious, malicious, or are subservient to the whims of unconscious, self-serving, unenlightened, thoughts and behaviors, we will be subject to unpleasant outcomes. The results will not be in harmony with universal law or our ultimate good.

The quantum interpretation of these same thoughts would be an imposition of adversity applied to the system of thoughts of an individual. The loss of the vision of health while being subjected to circumstances of distraction, such as an emotional distraction, is comparable to that of an athlete losing the image of competitive dominance because of an emotional distraction. This failure to "keep an eye on the prize" typically results in failure. The focus of our attention (imaging exercises) and our belief that we will obtain excellent health, impress upon us an empowered optimum outcome. While we recover from illness of any sort, focusing on our own positive image through organized, affirmative thought is the key to its acquisition! Proverbs 23:7 reads, "As a man thinketh in his heart, so is he." Also, Job noted in Job 3:25, "What I feared has come upon me; what I dreaded has happened to me" (New International Version.) This latter verse represents the adverse outcome of focusing attention on what we dread or fear.

Your vision is the promise of what you shall one day be; your ideal is the prophecy of what you shall at last unveil.

—James Allen

These quotes explain the effects of thoughts on our existence, and the effect of being the quantum participant in the determinism of our lives. They also imply the power of the mental principle of transmutation—changing from one form to another form. We manifest this transmutation when we continually think of desired—or undesired—outcomes until they finally impose themselves in our lives.

This principle seems to be quite straightforward, but it is not clearly understood, particularly when we consider the common chronic disease processes responsible for 70 percent of the health care budget ($2,500,000,000,000 plus per year and climbing). It would seem that our current health paradigm extols and advocates a path that leads to debilitating chronic health care woes.

We are the only country in the world to expend more than 16 percent of the gross domestic product on health care. The next closest competitor dispenses a mere 6 percent. That's a lot of money to spend without even being in the top thirty in terms of overall outcomes.

As I was discussing pain-healing issues with a new patient, the issues of thinking and thought became painfully evident to me. This patient's pain-healing issues resulted from moderately severe degenerative arthritis, as well as problems related to peripheral vascular disease and peripheral neuropathy (nerve damage). The source of his peripheral neuropathy and vascular disease was his longstanding diabetes, which itself was due to his longstanding morbid obesity and self-indulgent lifestyle. The degenerative arthritis was related to underlying osteoporosis from vitamin D deficiency, hypogonadism, and a history of tobacco abuse. The patient's reflection on the causality of his pain was, "It's not my fault!"

Now, I'm not always as confrontational as I was with this patient, but the process of using these laws necessitates understanding how our thoughts, based on a correct and adequate knowledge foundation, produce our health outcomes. So, my "gentle" discussion about this young man's eating habits, two-packs-per-day smoking habit, diabetes, and hypercholesterolemia detailed how his thinking (misinformed though it might be) and ensuing nutritional and lifestyle habits had resulted in his marginal health.

The education our team subsequently provided by compassionate discussions, as well as directed imaging, meditation on health, and biofeedback training imparted a knowledge base that was adequate enough to alter his thinking paradigm, and he successfully created a new image of health.

Quality of Thought as a Determinant of the Law

The infinite law of thinking in health is a critical spring boarding point of the universal laws, telling us it is our ruling state of mind (generating our beliefs, our attitudes, and so forth) that determines our lifetime experiences, and therefore, for our purposes, our health. What we believe, from an informed perspective, is what we will see insofar as our health is concerned. Or, more simply stated, what we consistently think about in terms of our health will manifest.

We should not presume that a thirty-minute perusal of the problem (or even thirty hours for that matter) on Web MD or "Dr. Google" is an adequate enlightenment to the current thought and practice on a health topic. While the information on any given subject may seem straightforward and easily comprehended, the best outcome may only result from fine-tuning with optimization of all parameters for the individual by a gifted and experienced practitioner. This is often the culmination of some trial and error depending on the complexity of the individual and the health care issue(s) at hand.

Even more so, caution must be given to the interpretation of any clinical trial work, particularly when we know through history that misinterpretations and generalizations have garnered adverse outcomes for the population at large in the past. As an example, the "food pyramid" advised by the FDA until about two years ago has now been changed considerably.

This is the conundrum and perplexity of misguided thought—a poor belief structure will give us poor results. The example of the old food pyramid that was erroneously conceived to avoid cholesterol and saturated fats was not in harmony with the universal good (not as intended for the good of mankind). We have, therefore, reaped the results of this misinterpretation of the data in the form of childhood diabetes and an epidemic of obesity along with the multiple complications of both of these diseases along with more heart disease. It is, therefore, only when our thoughts coincide with, or are synchronized to, those of universal good that they may then work well for the individual. This is a process of trial and error that will yield substantial benefit so long as it conforms to the universal good.

Your vision of health for yourself needs to be harmonious with, and can be pursued in the light of, what is universally accepted as good. Are physicians always correct in this regard? Clearly not. But as physicians and their patient-partners work conscientiously together to achieve an optimum health image, physicians will be able to provide the counsel of mentorship necessary to minimize deviations and errors of interpretation of the available information.

> *When we change our thinking for the better, we automatically change our lives for the better. … A change of thought must precede every change in the life (health) and in the affairs of man, when our intention becomes reconciled or cooperative with the universal (God's) intentions, then we become an expression of that good. This is working with the law.*
> —Raymond Holliwell, author of *Working with the Law: 11 Truth Principles for Successful Living*

Your Empowered Medicine Cabinet

Visualize Your Health

Conceptualize and write down at least twenty different health characteristics that describe your successful optimized healthy image.

While thinking about your list, you may want surround yourself with any objects, people, locations, events, and activities that enhance your image and feelings of success.

Occasionally, this exercise presents some challenges for my patient-partners, so I give some additional guidelines here to assist in this imaging process. It is possibly somewhat easier to subject the creative image to a number of more specific criteria. The most important criteria in the effort to create an image that will assist our patient-partners' efforts to empower and guide them toward successful completion are Form, Feeling, and Function.

Form is the external appearance that we perceive will best represent our empowered healthy image. This must be clearly delineated by the necessary metrics that define optimum health acquisition and bodily dimensions. For example, we must not acquiesce to a physical appearance that perpetuates poor health and chronic disease. Minimizing total body fat to 18 percent for a woman, and 15 percent for a man, however, assists in optimizing potential health span and longevity according to current population based data.

Feeling is the second parameter that needs exacting attention, as many of us have adapted to multiple restrictions in our lifestyles. We are like the frog in the hot water. If we heat the water slowly, the frog rarely attempts escape from the pot. If, however, the frog is dropped into the preheated water, he will immediately jump out to avoid being cooked. We have amazing reserve, but the progressive restrictions we impose upon ourselves are the lifestyle compromises that an optimized integrative approach will recover if the image is correct. Focusing on the sense of well-being that we had as young adults or teenagers often will help us find the descriptive vocabulary of the optimized health image we are looking for.

Lastly, and possibly most importantly, the ***function*** of the diverse organs that assist us in accomplishing the activities of our lives is key. Mental and cognitive function, sensory function, cardio-respiratory, digestive, kidney, hematologic, immune, musculoskeletal functions are all critical to being our best. Delineating optimum capabilities for all of these in the image of successful health assists in the optimization process.

Take a few moments to sit back, close your eyes, and create the image of your optimized health and lifestyle. This is the just the first step in acquiring your empowered health outcome. When you are ready, complete this exercise on the following form. Be mindful to avoid using negative terms such as no, not, without, don't, free of, and so forth. For example, instead of writing, "I feel pain free" or "I can walk without pain," write, "I feel comfortable" or "I can walk with ease." A few additional useful guidelines to the creation of statements for the successful image is to make them brief, in the present tense, the subject stated as first person, and make them assertively affirmative. (eg I am_____, I can _____, I have _____, I _____, I love to_____, and so forth). Lastly the use of objective measurements that serve as the arbiter of success are quite useful. They establish a quantitative endpoint at which celebrations may occur (e,g,. I can run a mile in seven minutes).

FORM (Physical appearance)	
Example: My body is strong	*Example: I move gracefully*

FEELING (Emotion)	
Example: I feel confident	*Example: I love my body*

FUNCTION **(What you can do)**	
Example: I run a mile in 8 minutes	*Example: I practice mediation and yoga daily*

CHAPTER 3

The Infinite Law of the Empowered Perspective and Health

A substantial challenge to our success is making sense of the origin of our problems. Very often, the source of a medical problem or symptom can be traced back to multiple factors. Those factors are not always the result of definable hereditary issues, but more often derive from self-inflicted stress or misguided good intentions.

A good example is diabetes. This multifactorial chronic disease originates from inadequate blood glucose control by the hormone insulin, potentially for a multitude of reasons. Simply, we either don't have enough insulin to effectuate control, or the quantity available is incapable of exercising its role. Insofar as the current diabetes epidemic is concerned, we have challenged our bodies abilities by overindulgence in the carbohydrate-rich nutritional lifestyles advocated by the FDA until their recommendations were superseded by the new food pyramid, which was premiered in 2014. Even the American Diabetes Association's recommended diet remains carbohydrate laden to this day. Who is minding the store here?

I discontinued administering these toxic nutritional regimens years ago, and as a result can no longer enumerate the complete resolutions of abnormal hemoglobin A1C levels amongst my patient population. (The A1C test measures the average blood sugar over a four-month period of time.) Additionally, the elimination of oral hypoglycemic medications and insulin saved these patients tens of thousands of dollars in pharmaceutical costs, just by the simple elimination of inappropriate foods from the nutritional lifestyle. No insulin, no oral medications, nothing but a modified nutritional lifestyle and—voilà!—proper adequate glucose control by the body!

When we eat carbohydrates, rapidly climbing blood glucose levels cause the release of endorphins and serotonin, which have calming, mood enhancing effects. From a practical perspective, this is self-sabotaging in times of moodiness. We refer to this as "comfort food" and use it therapeutically when our moods suffer. We consume comfort food to compensate for loneliness, sadness, depression, guilt, or other negative feelings caused by stressful and emotional situations. The withdrawal process from the mood-enhancing effects of neurotransmitters, such as serotonin, beta-endorphins, dopamine, and norepinephrine, can be quite difficult for some patients. It is in understanding this perilous "withdrawal" hormonal environment of the body that the mind-body directed imaging techniques and biofeedback we use at Infinite Health truly find a home.

As such, when we consider the infinite law of thinking in health, in this setting, it is easily understood that deviation of our thoughts outside of the known useful nutritional pathways will only create unwanted or unhealthy physical attributes, such as obesity and diabetes. These conditions ultimately generate further medical problems and compromise quality of life and health-span. The converse also holds true. By virtue of our quantum conscious intent as we maintain consistent thoughts on those qualities and benefits gained by a healthy nutritional lifestyle, we will unfold a consistently beneficial environment within our bodies, and will then reap the benefits of these ideas.

We must inform ourselves of the true nature of our undesirable health challenges. To do this, most of us need assistance and a plan that allows us to be the active, empowered participant implementing positive change. We do this by using available information resources, and by working with a physician or adequately trained health care practitioners who are well versed in comprehensive integrative care. This type of transformational mentorship allows us to find the sources of counterproductive behavior along with the limiting beliefs that have spawned them. These practitioners become our productive teachers of transformation and successful empowerment. They instill the type of thinking that ultimately yields a force of change for the better. (Remember that our thoughts are impacting our outcomes in this quantum reality). Empowered thought is a force that enables us to change for the better and to reap the great health we all deserve.

As we place more focus on the continued contemplation of healthy outcomes, we are directing the constructive quantum energy of belief or power of intention. This produces an effect of constructive beneficial change in the observed environment. In the setting of change, this represents the transmutation of energy to a productive rather than a destructive change.

We are always thinking, so it is important that the power or force of our thinking remains organized, disciplined, and constructive to yield a productive outcome. Misguided hearsay or meandering anecdotes frequently infuse the medical literature. Awareness of their use in the literature of the many pseudo-medical products permeating the Internet and the "wellness" marketplace help us to make wiser choices.

Additionally, the monkey brain is mischievous and may plant deviously contrary images in the mind. These images, most often the construct of ignorance, are produced just as readily as the healthy ones if our focus remains fixed on them. A constructive personalized plan prepared by a proficient practitioner of integrative medicine is probably the most productive initiative to pursue. Supervision by a transformational integrative physician provides the necessary accountability that improves the success of optimized health manifestation.

This simply means that all of us have the ability, by controlling our thoughts and their content, and therefore our minds, and the participation of our minds, to control the outcomes of our lives and health. So when we eat the deep-fried chicken, we shouldn't necessarily expect to avoid the stroke or acute coronary syndrome. Additionally, as our thoughts continue to focus on our successful health image and its benefits, our conscious self-awareness emits an energy that, with the continuous involvement of subconscious forces, attracts similar energies, vibrations, and thoughts; this is followed by a cascade of events and actions resulting in the desired outcome … great health! As we remain open-minded and receptive about the ultimate benefit of our collaborative interventions, our efforts will likely produce greater benefit than anticipated.

For those of us who are challenged by certain health-related issues, the participation in a structured program designed to provide guided imaging and biofeedback can also be very helpful. Guided imagery is a mind-body technique in which a trained practitioner guides the patient-partner in generating specific mental images designed to engage each of the senses. Biofeedback, which, according to Wikipedia is "… the process of gaining greater awareness of many physiological functions primarily using instruments that provide information on the activity of those same systems, with a goal of being able to manipulate them at will. These two scientifically proven complementary techniques, combined with patient education, as well as programmed behavior modification coursework in a supportive compassionate environment generates the best outcome. This type of program generates consistent empowered thinking and is like a beacon emitting a sort of homing signal for the desired outcome—or something even better. The most subtle of efforts mentally provides the desired outcome by virtue of the effects of empowering thought and belief on your life.

When we discipline ourselves to organize the thinking process around those thoughts that give rise to our single purposeful health end game, our minds can make easy work of achieving that vision by effectuating change on the system. It is only in finalizing the vision and in committing to the expected positive change that we powerfully extract the desired transformational destiny. The quality of our end product is the result of the quality and focus of our beliefs (thinking), vision, and effort, regardless of the point of departure.

On a more practical level, our thoughts should be addressed on two levels:

Level 1: Current Thinking

What is our current health-related reality? As individuals, in each area of challenge to our well-being, we must isolate the thoughts that may be impediments to healing and improvement. More importantly we must, at every given moment, maintain an image of our optimized health outcome, particularly if we are starting from a level of deficiency. This means that we must isolate the negative thoughts and beliefs we routinely foster in terms of our diagnoses, anticipated outcomes, and our treatment regimens and replace them with the positive images of our desired outcomes. Negative thoughts and beliefs have the potential to aggravate medical conditions by virtue of the type of physiologic stress responses our body has to them. These limiting thoughts and beliefs are important because they are the reflection of the anticipated outcomes for health communicated to the quantum matrix that establishes health and health span.

The perception of our health contributes to recreate our health reality by clearly focusing on the adequacy and veracity of each diagnosis we accept. From something as straight forward as a bone fracture, to the complexity of a multiple end-organ autoimmune disease such as systemic lupus erythematosus, our perception of possibilities realigns the efforts we are willing to provide to bring about change. Once the inventory of health issues is completed, and for many of us it may seem unending, the vision for fresh outcomes must be created. It is only then that we may begin feeding these images with our earnest effort and belief.

Level 2: Old Thinking

This represents many of those limiting beliefs instilled in our subconscious minds that may be holding us back from a better outcome. It is important to understand the limiting beliefs we harbor, which may or may not be of our own lifetime experiences such as parental and societal influences among others. And it's important to understand that each represents the equivalent of a ball and chain. Their very existence affects every effort we make to improve, and may be sabotaging our present and future health. In my practice, the goal is to provide patient-partners with tools that make certain their thoughts are their most fervent allies in the creation of good health. The exercises that we dispense are specifically designed to facilitate empowered self-realization and remove the limits that may have been innocently imposed by surroundings when our patient-partners were very young or that they acquired during their lifetimes.

Trip Goolsby, MD & LeNae Goolsby, JD

Guided Imagery in Medicine, Motivational Techniques, and Therapeutic Improvement

The infinite law of thinking and its principal benefits have been progressively evaluated and incorporated into occidental medicine over the past thirty or forty years. Doctor Herbert Benson made some of the pioneering studies that led to a less hesitant acceptance of these techniques by conventional physicians. Since that time, and even more so recently, clinical trial work incorporating a mind-body component to the comparison sampling cohort (guided imagery, meditation, motivational enhancement, among others) has objectively demonstrated significant improvement in outcomes.

Guided imagery is qualified as a directed program of thoughts or mental images and suggestions that enhance relaxation and focus on a desired outcome or state of being. This is often done using auditory programming and, on occasion, associated visual subliminal complementary video. Remember the response of the central nervous system to distress? Many of the improvements noted in clinical trial work in many areas can be related to enhanced relaxation and/or an improved sense of well-being. Guided imagery then engages, through activation of the central nervous system, all of the senses. The body, clueless as it is, "assumes" the sensory input originates from external sources and responds accordingly. Many of the directed imaging techniques use auditory enhancements in an effort to synchronize brainwave activity at a level that enhances relaxation and subconscious imprinting. Some have even demonstrated improved function of the immune system, when that condition is studied as the parameter of response.

I routinely appreciate improved participation with directed imagery techniques that use binaural auditory brainwave methodologies (brainwave entrainment). There are also visual subconscious programs that incorporate brain wave modulations to enhance therapeutic interventions. Studies have been successful in demonstrating improved outcomes in many areas, including, most notably, pain reduction, stress reduction for any type of stress-related disorder, and hypertension. In fact, dr. Benson's initial studies of the effects of meditation on disease processes began with a focus on hypertension. Additional positive outcomes have been observed in studies for congestive heart failure, acute coronary syndrome, stroke prevention and rehabilitation, obesity, smoking cessation, and the treatment of other substance addictions such as narcotics and alcohol. Lastly, anxiety, depression, and panic disorders all respond more significantly with the use of a mind-body component.

It seems that medical professionals and patients alike are confirming the utility of the infinite law of thinking. We are able to enhance and balance our lives significantly by simply thinking about how and what we want in our lives while maintaining a crisp, clear picture on conscious and subconscious levels.

Motivational techniques are currently being studied as an adjunct to optimized medical management in the setting of many disease processes. Although rigorous, objective parameters for physiologic end points or survival end points may be easily defined, those related to quality of life or more subjective parameters generally provide increased challenge, as they require an objective scaling. While these techniques garner positive outcomes, they may simply be related to the effect of "caring," which, nowadays, sadly, is often lacking. This caring is no longer, in my observation, a component of most patient-physician interactions. I would really like to blame the evolution of medical economics and health care delivery for this problem. It was, is, and ever shall be, however, the responsibility of the provider to provide care; thus, the dilemma.

In the current system, physicians are compensated more for their technical ability than for their compassion. Ultimately, when I say technical ability, I mean the ability to efficiently prescribe a pharmaceutical product or dispense a procedure. In contrast, in my experience, I have found that the physician's ability to impart the energy and vibration of caring, understanding, acceptance, as well as humor and happiness produces the most beneficial effect for the patient.

It would seem that William James was of a similar opinion in his day, as he studied to be a physician at Harvard but ultimately never practiced. He reflected about the use of pharmaceuticals: "My first reflections is that there is much humbug therein, and that, with the exception of surgery in which something positive is sometimes accomplished, a doctor does more by the moral effect of his presence on the patient and family, than by anything else."

It is, therefore, the thought of healing and health itself that physicians impress upon their minds that rules the day and provides the vision of what can be—hope, belief—for every patient. Likewise, the vision, image, or thought that we create with the assistance of our health care provider/coach/partner should be our empowered promise to ourselves. The optimized health we agree upon, with guidance, is the prediction of what we will eventually obtain. There will then be no compromise, and our minds will motivate us to the ultimate acquisition of this vision. The outcome we obtain is the quantum-based clinical effect accomplished by virtue of the partnership and combined effort—action over time and distance resulting from the energy of thought—of patient and clinicians together. This is integrative care.

From a transformational perspective, we are nurturing a clinical effect that results from the quantum clinical input of patient and practitioner. By this methodology, we are providing a means of empowered individual self-development and enlightenment using guidelines for personal success while at the same time directing the acquisition of extraordinary physical, spiritual, and intellectual health. The thinking that develops from these exercises and readings will guide the body to improved longevity while responding to the question: How do we make the best of our health during our time here on this physical plane?

Your Empowered Medicine Cabinet

Establish a Daily Meditation Practice

Daily meditation is proven to have many health benefits, such as the following:

- Lowers high blood pressure
- Lowers levels of blood lactate, which may reduce anxiety and anxiety attacks
- Decreases tension-related pain, such as tension headaches, insomnia, and joint issues
- Increases serotonin production, thereby improving mood and behavior
- Improves the immune system
- Increases energy levels
- Brings brainwave patterns into an alpha state that promotes self-healing
- Improves emotional stability
- Increases happiness levels
- Helps one gain clarity and peace of mind
- Sharpens the mind
- Reduces feelings of instability and being overwhelmed

Here's how to do it:

Ideally, we want to meditate twice a day for at least fifteen minutes each time. However, if our schedules are not conducive to meditating twice a day, we will still receive benefits by practicing once a day. The best times of the day to meditate are first thing in the morning upon waking and right before sleep at night.

The most frequent challenge when beginning to meditate is the wandering mind. This is natural and okay. The mind simply needs to be trained, and it is not necessary to become frustrated or discouraged if this process takes some time. When you become aware that your mind has wandered, simply redirect attention back to your breathing or your image of success for health. You will find in due time that your mind no longer wanders, and the fifteen minutes fly by.

Guided Meditation for Infinite Health

The following is a partial script from the group meditation classes offered by Infinite Health. You may use this guided mediation to assist you as well. When you are ready, find a soothing space to relax. You may sit in a comfortable position, or you may lie down.

Close your eyes.

Take a deep breath to the count of four. Hold it to a count of four, and release it to a count of six.

Again, take a deep breath in to a count of four, hold to a count of four, and release to a count of six.

And one more time—deep breath in to a count of four, hold to a count of four, and release to a count of six.

Now imagine that you are at your favorite location—that place that offers you the most peace, the most relaxation. This may be the beach, a cabin in the mountains, or even your own back porch in the still of the morning, perhaps watching the sunrise. Whatever place brings you the most peace is good. This is your private space. Your time is your own, you are free from all responsibilities in this moment. All is well, and it is safe and good for you to be in this space for this time.

Fully engage all of your senses. Notice the colors of the scenery: the yellow brilliance of the sun, the baby blue sky, the glittering ocean, or the vibrant green of the leaves on the trees and in the fields.

Tune into the sounds that are around you. Notice if you hear birds singing, waves rushing into the shore and back out again, or the rustling of the leaves, perhaps.

Notice how you feel. Is there a breeze gently teasing your hair? Do you feel the warmth of the sun on your face? How does the ground feel beneath your feet?

Notice the aromas around you. Do you smell the crispness of the air or the scent of wildflowers, or perhaps something else?

Spend a few minutes here, breathing in and out deeply and slowly, in the place of serenity, security, and where all is well.

When you are ready, notice that, off in the distance, someone is walking toward you. This person seems familiar, but you are not sure if you know who it is. As this person gets closer and closer, you see he or she is smiling and appears to be genuinely happy and at peace.

And as this person comes up to you and stands in front of you, you realize that this person is you. This is you in your most vibrant, most energetic, and most healthy physical state.

Notice how this ideal version of you appears in your ideal toned, fit, and youthful-looking body. Your skin is glowing; your hair is shiny and healthy. You are smiling, at peace with yourself, with others, and the world.

See yourself and this ideal, infinitely healthy version of yourself meld together and become one.

Now notice how you feel in your ideal state of health.

How much more energy do you have?

Notice how easy it is to move, to walk, to run, and even jump.

Notice how full of peace and joy you are.

Notice how wonderful, happy, and in love with yourself and with you life you are when you are in your optimized state of physical, emotional, mental, and spiritual health.

Stay in this space for a few minutes, breathing deeply, in and out.

Feel and know that this is who you already are.

And when you are ready to open your eyes, you may do so.

Elongate your back, take a deep breath in and release it. Reach your hands up to the sky, then out to the sides, and join them together in front of you.

And when you are ready, open your eyes.

CHAPTER 4

The Infinite Law of Supply in Health

Natalie is an upbeat, blonde, thirty-nine-year-old, obese woman brought in by her sister to see if I could help with weight loss and some "other" issues that were not clearly delineated prior to the first visit. She was, in fact, a cancer survivor who had undergone a bone marrow transplant for acute leukemia about eleven years earlier. A number of other issues had developed in association with the immune response from her transplant. These included chronic conjunctivitis, hypothyroidism, and arthritis. Prior to seeing me, she was being treated for chronic pain, depression, and anxiety. Treatment included multiple antidepressant medications, antianxiety medications, as well as narcotic pain medications. Her anxiety and depression had been aggravated more recently by the murder-suicide of her mother by her stepfather.

Natalie's primary focus was on her weight, hormonal balancing, as well as issues related to her insomnia, anxiety, and depression. Although hormonal balancing was previously attempted with an oral regimen, by her prior physician, the hormones prescribed were not bioidentical in nature. Bioidentical hormones have the identical molecular form as those produced in the human body. She did not recall any benefit from that hormonal regimen. At the same time, her depression and anxiety were being treated by the administration of a selective serotonin reuptake inhibitor (SSRI) with moderately effective results, albeit with a significant concomitant weight gain.

Natalie also had a two-pack-per-day smoking habit and had no intention of quitting that habit prior to her first visit at Infinite Health. Because of her mood deficit and inability to obtain significant improvement with the regimen prescribed by her primary physician, she had lost hope for significant improvement; that is, until her sister insisted that Natalie come to see me.

Natalie's evaluations disclosed inadequate hormone levels for estradiol, testosterone, thyroid, progesterone, as well as other hormone precursors. Her total cholesterol and LDL cholesterol (the bad cholesterol) were quite elevated. Her blood work was sound, however, except for a mild macrocytic (enlarged red blood cells) anemia.

Her loss of hope had registered on a deeper level. Natalie was unable to see herself improving on any front—until we discussed her goals for positive outcomes. As she initiated the Infinite Health program, one of the key empowerment techniques we used to reinforce her successful involvement was the creation of an image of ideal health and well-being. As instructed, she was to focus on this desired image of her well-being and improve upon it, as she felt appropriate throughout the course of care. This image is effectively created by the patient and incorporated into the brainwave-entrainment-assisted guided imaging meditations throughout the healing process. Natalie created her initial image shortly after completing her preliminary evaluations, and she has updated them on several occasions. Enhanced by our infinite health intention board exercise, her anticipated outcome now revolves around a much more vibrant and active young woman wearing size eight clothes, down from the initial size of sixteen, who no longer smokes and is actively involved with her social contacts and community.

Although it is too soon to tell at the time of this writing, she is showing great promise in fulfilling her imagined self by having already discontinued her smoking habit, and having lost twenty-five percent of her desired weight loss objective. She is also responding nicely to her bioidentical hormone replacement therapy and hormone supplementation, which has allowed for the cessation of her SSRI. Her demeanor is significantly more affirmative because her focus is now fixed squarely on her imaged goals.

In discussions with our patient-partners, we use the universal law of supply to empower patient choices related to their desired health outcomes. This is done in the context of their imaging brainwave entrainment sessions. These sessions are recommended twice daily, morning and evening. They serve to reinforce the thought process that drives an ongoing desire to achieve the imaged goals. This resembles the approach of Napoleon Hill in his seminal text on business success, *Think and Grow Rich*, which has guided so many businesswomen and men to success.

The law of supply states that whatever we desire and believe in our heart is ours. The simple fact that we have the desire and belief is the effect of the preexisting cause. The cause is that our desire exists for us already at the time that the demand or desire occurs. Our outcome is available to us by virtue of our earnest desire, and is subsequently provided to us. The key to the law of supply is belief in the existence of whatever is desired. We are continually using this law. As long as we believe in the outcome and continue to desire and expect its appearance in our lives, it shall be so. The universal law of supply tells us that the essential substance of every imaginable good exists, and that our desires, thoughts, and images serve as indicators that the good from this essential substance is already available to us.

Jesus said, "Ask, and it shall be given to you; seek, and ye shall find; knock, and it shall be opened unto you" (Matthew 7:7 KJV). Here, the Bible relates the notion that believing in the results is tantamount to achieving them, and in so saying, it tells us that we are never meant to be satisfied with our current state in life. This does not mean we are meant to be frustrated with the conditions of our lives. Although this happens when we misunderstand the nature of challenges and obstacles that occur. Rather, we are always moving forward into new conditions of enlightenment, knowledge, and physical being, and these provide us with new perspectives on our lifetime conditions, and from those we acquire new desires and better goals and outcomes.

Jesus also said, "What things soever ye desire, when ye pray, believe that ye receive them, and ye shall have them" (Mark 11:24 KJV).

We can be reasonably confident in that outcome because it already exists. It exists in our future as we have defined it: Believe it, then you will see it. (Of course, a negative outcome can materialize the same way if we focus on the negative!) The supply is always ready and available for us. Whatever we want is there for us; it can be no other way. We should expect no less when it comes to our health, regardless of the perceived distance between where we are and where we want to go. When we perceive that we need a better outcome for our health, that good health is there for us by virtue of a never-ending supply. That supply may simply be accessed by our belief and fervent intent to realize its existence. (Remember Fran?)

What is the sequence of events that activates the appearance of the supply? It is simply the appearance of the demand. That said, the active thought of the desire, the idea (belief) of an improved condition in our health is evidence that the supply exists. Our inspired idea for better physical, mental, and emotional health creates that material supply in our future. We must, however, create the demand. It is to our misfortune that, in most cases, we are not aware that we have control of the machine that produces the supply at all times. That, however, is our incorrect thinking. Our thoughts are the architects of our health, and we must consider them as such.

Likewise, to our detriment, our trusted advisors and health care professionals, in a majority of cases, are keen to dwell and focus on adverse outcomes. This is so you won't be disappointed if the outcome is, indeed, adverse. The advice that we are offered in this setting of lack and fear does not allow us to focus on the creation of an image of positive desire.

> *At the outset, let us realize that the material world in which we live is a sphere of effects and the behind these effect is a world of causes. Then recognize that when you desire any particular effect, it is because that [this] specific "good" is already in existence in the sphere of causes. Then recognize that when you desire any particular effect, this desire is an appearance [in your consciousness] of an underlying cause.*
>
> —Raymond Holliwell

As long as the thoughts are creating the desired (as opposed to undesired) demand, the supply has already been created, and it flows toward the positive end result. It is important not to lose track of, or weaken, our connection to the healthy positive image by becoming distracted by worry over, or doubt about, the final result. If such thoughts come, simply brush them away, without judgment, and return your focus to the desired outcome. Relaxation and confidence in the final outcome is necessary to accomplishing the simple task of accessing the supply. Relaxation and focus is part of the methodology used in the morning and evening imaging sessions along with brainwave entrainment guided imaging sessions. These sessions transform our thoughts and minds into magnets for the optimum outcome we are seeking.

If our thoughts are consistently focused on sickness and disease, we are continuing to prepare for and demand sickness from the infinite supply. An example of this would be thinking primarily about arranging and organizing the medicines we use to treat the sicknesses we have. The universe responds to all our thoughts: "Oh, yes, we certainly have more of that for you!"

Lapsing into thoughts about "my pain," "my swelling," "my weight," "my congestive heart failure," "my smoking," "my this and my that" will accomplish no more than a decreased focus in the demand for good from the infinite supply. It is for this reason that our focus must be always upward to the best result we can conceive. This conception will, as I mentioned earlier, upon each small success, give rise to new perspectives of incremental benefit and even better outcomes as we advance.

We must, at all costs, ignore the negative self-talk and despairing thoughts of the naysayers as we pursue our best results. Our behavioral mind-body training program provides techniques to shift negative focus to positive, as does using associated biofeedback technologies.

Remember, focused thoughts of our best possible outcome activate the infinite supply. They also subconsciously activate the body's organs to improve our health. In the event you feel you are having overwhelmingly destructive thoughts, take a meditation break and renew your imaging. Reflect on your successes and activate your gratitude. These will give you a better perspective of the accomplishments you have attained, and will help you know you are achieving your ideal. Additionally, using biofeedback or other contemplative mindfulness resources will serve to reorient our focus before the adverse and stressful thoughts effectively gather enough momentum to attract nefarious outcomes.

If we truly have the desire for better health, in whatever form or domain we perceive, it is because the desired effect of good health already exists for us. Although this may sound somewhat backwards in its context, it is in fact in compliance with a number of scientific principles that were formulated in the early twentieth century by some little-known physicists—Einstein, Plank, Schrodinger, Bohr, and Heisenberg, with contributions and an addendum later added by Everett. All of these gentlemen were Nobel laureates in physics, with the exception of Everett.

The conclusions drawn from the respective works and theorems of Einstein, Plank, Schrodinger, Bohr, Heisenberg, et al., gave rise to changes in the paradigm of thought. They proved that we are no longer simple observers of the world (and thereby, I say, our health). We are, in fact, participants in the outcomes, affecting the very stuff our universe and lives are made of. Not that this concept is really new. Religious and philosophic masters have long been aware of the impact of our thoughts and beliefs on our environment. Indeed, we have just read quotes from the New Testament and authors whose writings date from before the Nobel Laureate physicists determined the principles of quantum physics. And there are so many more. It took only a few thousand years for the scientific community to confirm the intuitive results!

The act of us simply looking at our world—projecting the feelings and beliefs that
we have as we focus our awareness on the particles that the universe is made of—
changes those particles as we are looking.
—Gregg Braden, author of *The Spontaneous Healing of Belief*

In 1957, Hugh Everett III presented his doctoral thesis in physics at Princeton. It was a resolution to certain problematic issues of quantum physics theory. At the same time, it created the scientific explanation of an infinite number of synchronous past and future time lines and universes. His many-worlds interpretation of quantum mechanics suggests that any possible future and/or past time lines may coexist simultaneously with the present one. These time lines are separated only by the differences of decisions we make at the moment of occurrence, and are influenced by virtue of the thoughts and beliefs we have about the situation or the subject we are considering at the time.

For our empowered health purposes, this means any outcome we desire is possible from the time we believe we may attain it. Although the most-effective means to functionally improve our individual systems have yet to be completely outlined, the modalities we are pursuing, in the context of my empowered motivational medicine program, are proving to be effective, particularly in the setting of chronic diseases. We are potentially intensifying the effectiveness of conventional medicine approaches by facilitating compliance with the quantum nature of the universal laws, and the theoretical nature of the laws of quantum physics. These quantum concepts were often taken up by Jesus in his discussions with his disciples. For example, he said, "Blessed are those who have not seen and yet have believed." (John 20:29 New International Version).

The implication of this usage is that the blessings of belief are obtained in the absence of visualization. We will see and obtain that in which we believe—the blessings of our desires. Ergo, quantum mechanics were discussed in the first century AD.

As we choose to create a life of empowered health, our vision, imaging, and thoughts become the tools that impose direction toward the desired outcome. In a quantum sense, the observers (us) decide what form of health they will have by virtue of their fundamental beliefs and continued focus on the desired result. This is our energy of thought taking shape ultimately as the image of the excellent health we desire.

Your Empowered Medicine Cabinet

Create Your Infinite Health Intention Board

Practicing visualization and setting intentions are two of the most powerful mind exercises we can do. According to Rhonda Byrne's popular book, *The Secret*, the law of attraction is forming our entire life experience through our core beliefs, our thoughts, and our feelings, whether we are conscious of it or not. When we visualize, we emit a powerful vibratory frequency that brings to us whatever we focus on.

Visualization, when combined with setting our intention, is a powerful process that is proven to effectuate our desires. In fact, this process is used by Olympic athletes because it successfully aids them in their ability to improve their success. *Psychology Today* reports that the brain patterns activated when a weightlifter actually lifts heavy weights are also similarly activated when the lifter just imagines (visualizes) lifting the weights.

Create a sacred space that illustrates what you want. This will actually bring your desires to life as your energy flows where your attention goes. Then create an intention board—or vision board— and place it where you will see it often. Whenever you look at it, you will be engaging in mini-visualization processes throughout the day.

There is no right or wrong way to create your intention board. It is all about pulling together images and words that inspire you, that help you maintain your focus on the optimized infinitely healthy body and life that you desire.

When selecting the images for your intention board, choose pictures and quotes that resonate with your highest vision for your health and life. The idea of having, or being, or stepping into the picture ideally will evoke a positive emotional feeling.

For example, if you dream of one day having a home with a bedroom view of the ocean, choose a picture of that home, or of that bedroom view of the ocean. Step into the picture and imagine how awesome and amazing it would feel to wake up every morning to see a beautiful crystal-blue ocean, an orange-and-pink sunrise, and to smell and feel of the early morning salty air whipping through your unbrushed morning bed head.

Perhaps for the vision of optimized health, you will choose a picture of someone else in an optimized state of health, or a picture of yourself when you were at your healthiest. Step into that picture and imagine how much energy you will have, how good you will feel, and all the wonderful adventures you will experience when you realize that perfect state of health.

Many people may have difficulty even beginning to know what it is that they desire for their lives. If you're thinking, "Yeah! That's me! I have no idea where to begin!" No worries. It is absolutely okay.

To help you gain clarity so that you begin to set your intentions toward your infinite health and life, answer the following questions without over thinking the answers. After you have answered, ask yourself, "Now, what would be even better than that?" Push the limits of your imagination.

- If you could have a life beyond your wildest imagination, what would that look like? Think about where are you living, whom you are living with (or without). What does your typical day look like? What are you doing that brings you joy?
- How do you feel when you first wake up in the morning? What activities, practices, and/or things would help you feel that way every day?
- When you were a child what did you want to be when you grew up? Why? What can you do today that makes you feel the same way?

You intuitively know what resonates, what feels good to you, and what does not. Trust your feelings as you begin to select your pictures and quotes for your intention board. Here are some quotes that I like:

- "The secret to having it all is believing that you already do." —Source unknown
- "Our intention creates our reality." —Dr. Wayne Dyer
- "Create the highest grandest vision possible for your life because you become what you believe." —Oprah Winfrey
- "Whatever you hold in your mind on a consistent basis is exactly what you will experience in your life." —Anthony Robbins, author of *Awaken the Giant Within*
- "If you are working on something you really care about, you do not have to be pushed— the vision pulls you." —Steve Jobs

Your Intention Board on Nitrous Oxide (NOS)

Admittedly, everything I know about NOS I learned from *The Fast and the Furious* film series, which, as I understand it, essentially is that, when Brian O'Connor pushes the red NOS button, as he's drag racing to the finish line, his car accelerates so fast that he nearly gets whiplash, and Brian loves it.

Adding intentional affirmations to your daily intention board envisioning process, while honing in on your internal emotional personal guidance system, is like adding Brian O'Connor– grade NOS to your car. You will begin to allow that which you desire to come to you even faster.

Everything is energy vibrating at various levels. Our thoughts, our words, and our emotions are also energy vibrating at various levels. When we choose to think positively, when we choose to speak positively, and when we choose to feel happy, joyful, blissful, and loving, regardless of what is appearing in our life experience at any given moment, we are choosing to be in alignment with our heart's desire, and that, my friends, is how we open the door for that which we desire to show up for us.

Ideally, you should take a few minutes in the morning right before you get out of bed and in the evening right before you go to sleep to meditate on your intention board, getting into the feeling of the symbols you have selected for the life you desire. You should repeat affirmations that support your intentions. For example, for more energy and a healthier body, your intentional affirmations could be:

- I am so thankful and grateful for the energy I have.
- I have more than enough energy.
- I am so thankful and grateful for the health that I have, and I know that I am already healed. I am already whole.

Thinking intentionally, which is supported by your intention board, helps you to speak intentionally, which is supported by your intentional affirmation statements. Both of these practices will help you feel lighter and more joyful, and this opens doors so you can let in whatever you desire when it shows up for you.

Once your board is completed, take a picture of it and share it with us via our Infinite Health FaceBook page located at https://www.facebook.com/LiveTheInfiniteLife/.

Here is one of LeNae's intention boards:

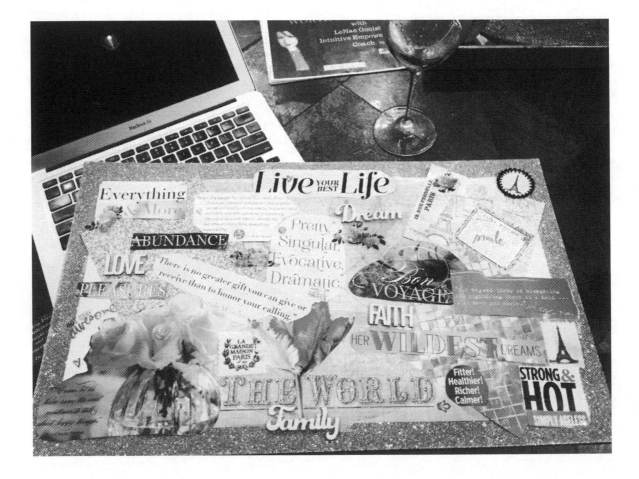

CHAPTER 5

The Infinite Law of Attraction in Health

Steven is a forty-nine-year-old obese male who came in for an evaluation of the persistent pain in his lower left leg, the result of a left hip fracture and fracture of his heel bone after an automobile accident. This accident was the cause of severe degenerative disease in his left knee, which required a total knee replacement approximately eight months prior to his first visit with me.

In addition to his knee pain, Steven was an inveterate smoker of about thirty years, at a pack to a pack and a half a day, and had a mild to moderate case of chronic obstructive pulmonary disease. He also suffered from mild hypertension, fatigue, mild cognitive dysfunction, moodiness, irritability, decreased libido, erectile dysfunction, and seasonal allergies.

Although Steven had been following a routine schedule of visits with his family physician, that physician declined to manage the knee pain he was having, and ignored Steven's repeated attempts to discuss his significant other health issues; he refused to pursue the necessary evaluations required to asses the origins of Steven's health concerns, choosing instead to only prescribe Steven with blood pressure medication. It is unsurprising then that the State of Louisiana sought fit to declare Steven as a disabled person, incapable of re-entering the workforce.

Steven sought out our pain-healing program following the recommendation of another patient, who had experienced significant improvements through working with us. (I prefer the term *pain healing* to *pain management* because the focus is *resolving* the pain, using all effective therapeutic interventions over time. Rather than simply using medication in an attempt to control pain, the focus is to minimize any and all causes and aggravators of the pain.) But, by the time Steven came to see me, he was interested only in obtaining pain medication for his knee. He was completely disinterested in further enquiry into whether his condition could be improved by techniques other than narcotic medications. He requested that I simply continue his 80–120 milligrams of oxycodone daily, along with nonsteroidal anti-inflammatory drugs and muscle relaxants.

Steven's initial evaluation disclosed significantly decreased testosterone levels, a moderately decreased bone density, a severe vitamin D deficiency, and biochemistries compatible with early adrenal dysfunction, as well as elevated inflammatory markers. Similarly, his estradiol level was found to be compatible with a high risk for coronary artery disease. His elevated inflammatory indices were, in all likelihood, related to his moderate obesity and pre-diabetic average blood glucose levels (A1C).

We advised him to follow our proprietary 4-Pillars Approach, which includes:

- An aggressive nutritional lifestyle modification;
- An advancing exercise regimen of nonimpact high-intensity interval aerobic and flexibility training;
- Hormonal and metabolic optimization, which included pharmacy-grade vitamin D supplements, testosterone, thyroid supplement optimization, along with other neutriceutical supplementation; and
- Mind-body techniques, including our "Empowered Medicine" coaching and biofeedback.

After four to six months, Steven's pain improved to the point where he no longer required the aid of a cane or other supportive device. His pain medications were significantly decreased to the simple use of a single 10-milligram hydrocodone preparation two to four times a day as needed with a muscle relaxant in the evenings on occasion. He likewise quit smoking within two months of initiating the program. His moodiness, cognitive dysfunction, erectile dysfunction, decreased libido, energy levels, and endurance all improved significantly as he positively responded to hormonal optimization. All metabolic endocrine and inflammatory parameters were in optimum ranges for the duration of his treatment.

What I found most enlightening was Steven's focus and desire to improve, after he realized he could. I see this occur frequently as improvements in the sense of well-being establish new thresholds of activity and well-being for my patients. Steven's meditative directed imaging and his intention to achieve his optimum outcome never faltered. He pursued the program directives as he received them and maintained the attitude of achievement as though his optimum outcome was a given.

Briefly stated, the law of attraction is "like attracts like." This is a thought philosophy that relates that whatever thoughts and desires we have, positive or negative, will produce like experiences in our health, as well as our overall lives. Our thoughts are energy, and these energetic desires, and/or belief messages of well-being effectuate the attraction of like energetic health outcomes.

In sum, the appearance of a positive or advantageous health outcome is dependent on the action of our thought energy—desire, intention, vision on the substance of supply ether/quantum field. What is important for us to remember is that we have the capacity, by virtue of our conceptual abilities—mind and executive brain function—to imprint our intentional content on the surrounding energy fields so that the fields may be effectively changed. By doing this, we may then receive the benefits of our creativity.

It is important and easy to understand this from a health standpoint. Why? Because our bodies are constantly remodeling themselves from our ideas, thoughts, intentions, as well as our actions. For example, with the simple intent to stop smoking, we create an entirely different epigenetic and subsequent intracellular environment, which begins the remodeling of all subsequent cells that are to be created from the existing ones. Knowing that the cells in our bodies turn over completely in about seven years—more or less depending on the organ—we are easily able to effectuate the product of our intent to attract excellent health (improve our breathing and prevent smoking-related lung disease), or not.

Interestingly, the philosophical background of the law of attraction dates far back into antiquity. It is also supported by current quantum physics, as we exposed here briefly in the chapter about the law of supply. The concept of the law of attraction was taken up prior to quantum physics confirmation in the 1800s by New Thought philosopher and healer, Phineas Quimby. When he was a younger man, and in spite of multiple traditional medical failures, Mr. Quimby apparently "healed" himself of tuberculosis. The use of his mind-body approach gained significant popular support and was coupled with the use of hypnotism.

New Thought authors and "healers" attributed many "dis-eases" to the negative emotional thought processes of fear, worry, stress, and/or any other negative thinking. That belief also postulated that healing and the maintenance of well-being are the result of positive thinking or "right" thoughts.

Health and disease avoidance are not the only results of this "new thinking" philosophy, which also includes wealth, relationships, and success, in virtually any domain. This same axiom is also known to be the basis of some of the best-selling personal development references of all time, such as *Think and Grow Rich* by Napoleon Hill.

> *Whatever the mind can conceive and believe, it can achieve.*
>
> —Napoleon Hill

If you desire something related to your health, it already exists. Your desire must then be paired with expectation (intent) in order to achieve the anticipated outcome.

> *Always rid yourself of desires in order to observe its secrets, but always allow*
> *yourself to have desires in order to observe its manifestations.*
>
> —Lao Tze, *Tao De Ching*

This means that, if we are free from desires, we have a sense of completeness and wholeness, but desires give rise to manifestations. So, if we can master our focus (attention) in the present, then we can define (expect or intend) what we will manifest (create and attract). Ultimately, from the individual perspective, this means we can manifest good for all through the desire and intent of good (excellent health acquisition). This obviously includes the good (excellent health) for oneself.

Desire can be defined as focused interest in or a longing or craving for something. Our empowered intentions for excellent health are effectively supported and reinforced by the individual desires that fuel them. If excellent health is defined uniformly in a population, then greater attention must be drawn by the individual to his or her desired outcome, and it must be colored into that uniqueness. Our desire must be drawn to our intent consistently and effectively by our unique continued effort.

To be sure, many people who have chronic health problems become consumed with *thoughts* of their disease. Their day-to-day existence is focused on the delivery of medication and on activities that may not be drawing them into better health. This type of focus leads to repeated actions and habits that are, in fact, detrimental to their good health. This is because the expectation and intention of having good health no longer enters the thought process routinely; neither is there any interest in focusing on good or improved health because of the all-encompassing need to organize the lifestyle around a multitude of "dis-ease" management issues. For example, I have many pain healing patients like Steven who focus only on their pain medication and refer to their pain and/or illness as if it was a loving pet. Another example includes the diabetic who is focused only on high blood sugar and the prescription medications necessary to control that high blood sugar. These patients' better interests would be served to focus on comfort and ease of function for the former, and excellent nutrient processing for the latter.

> *Never expect anything you do not want,*
> *and never desire a thing you do not expect.*
>
> —Raymond Holliwell

When we look at our current health care system, and the reactive delivery modalities that dominate the provision of care, the treatment received by the vast majority of patients is focused on speedy prescription delivery—symptom management—rather than comprehensive planning for long-term problem resolution. When physician interest and intent are centered on healing and facilitating excellent health and/or its acquisition, then we actually begin to see excellent health and its acquisition. If most providers no longer expect to see resolution and instead project a lack of desire to treat, a lack of intent to cure, or a lack of appropriate compassion to assist in true healing, how can patients even begin to attempt, on their part, to focus on a healthy resolution of their medical challenges? How indeed may the "trusting uneducated" change the thoughts that have become so ingrained in the collective mind as the "standard" of care? A critical example of this is the current dilemma of pain "management." If we are managing pain, then we are no longer interested in its resolution. Expectation, belief, and intent are at the forefront of the law of attraction. Expectation and intent are the active forms of belief in an outcome. Expectation is the strong belief that something will happen in the future. It is the anticipation of materialization, the feeling of hope with a belief of ultimate achievement, or intent. Desire connects us with the health we want; it draws our attention to the end result. And expectation—the energy that produces forward momentum—draws it to us.

The Sequencing Formula For An Empowered Health Destiny:

Thought and thinking lead to beliefs and action. And these actions reinforce the beliefs, which lead to new habits, which lead to new character traits, which lead to destiny!

The new thoughts and thinking that we acquire by virtue of our independent education plus that education provided to us by our healthcare team will help us create new, well-founded beliefs and actions. The actions necessary to attract this new health outcome are those actions that we take of our own volition, as well as those that our physicians may guide or empower us to effectuate. This guidance, with or without prescription medication, is the active component that further reinforces, or optimizes, the connection (attraction) with the imaged empowered health outcome we desire (destiny).

To desire is to expect; to expect is to achieve.

—Raymond Holliwell

This is an enormously important consideration for our health. When working with our physicians, we envision our recoveries from any chronic disease processes. Our positive expectations lead to conquest. If we desire the physique and health of a marathon runner, a sprinter, a bodybuilder, but in turn have little or no expectation of its acquisition, we are simply dreaming; we are not expecting the fruit of our desire. When our empowered actions implement our beliefs, it is then that we attract and accomplish our empowered health destiny.

One of the most important actions we are already taking is to create the image of our desired health outcome using the twice-daily brainwave entrainment meditations. This activity is similar to those used by professional athletes to achieve their greatest success in competition. And, yes, we are intensely training for our optimum health and longevity.

Consider the following biblical Old Testament narrative in 2 Kings 4:1–7, whereby a widow came to the prophet Elisha and told him that creditors were coming to take her sons to be slaves, so Elisha asked her what she had in her house. When she said she had nothing but a small pot of oil, Elisha told her to borrow empty vessels from her neighbors, and not to borrow just a few. When she had done that, he said she must go inside, shut her door, and pour oil from her pot into all of the vessels. She did this, and the oil stayed, and when she had filled the last one, she asked for another, but there was not another empty vessel in the house. She went out and told Elisha she had done as he had told her, and he told her to go and sell the oil, pay her debts, and live.

Notice the widow received only enough oil to fill the exact number of jars that she had collected, and then the oil stopped flowing. This is indicative of receiving what we expect to receive. By all means, push the limits of your imagination.

Your Empowered Medicine Cabinet

Your Infinite Health Intention Board—Double Dose

In the previous chapters, you began your daily meditation practice and created your Infinite Health Intention Board. You have also been spending five to ten minutes daily focusing on the symbols and representations of your "happy end result," really stepping into the feeling of having that optimized health and life you desire. Keep it up! You are doing an awesome job, so we are now going to take your focus on your intentions to the next level.

For the next several weeks, choose one to two items from your intention board and consciously look for references to them during your day. For example, if you desire to run in a marathon, begin to look for and notice runners and running gear and/or for running events to show up in your day. Perhaps you'll notice someone running along the side of the road; perhaps you'll notice people around you talking about running, or you might see running on television. As another example, you might have the word *joy* on your intention board. Begin to notice every time you see or hear the word *joy* in the day. Perhaps you are introduced to someone whose name is Joy, or you see the word *joy* on a billboard or in a magazine.

This "medicine" is designed to show you, from a practical perspective, that energy flows to where our attention goes. By beginning to consciously shift our focus to that which we desire, we begin to bring that which we desire into our experience, from health to loving relationships to wealth. Keep it light. Make it a game you play with yourself, and perhaps even get your children to play along as well. Keep us posted of your successes on our Facebook page.

CHAPTER 6

The Infinite Law of Receiving in Health

Roger is a thirty-eight year-old health fanatic who has been a patient-partner for several years now. He has few medical issues, aside from the recent challenges presented by his competitive need to win a bodybuilding event. That said, he was quite frustrated by his continuing inability to achieve the muscular definition and decreased body fat levels that would accommodate a competitive stature. Historically, this had not been an issue because, typically, some minor increased effort on his part in the gym would result in improved muscular tone and presentation. Now, however, he was not as inclined to pursue his customary exercise routines; neither was his ability up to his usual standard of endurance. These subtle changes took place over the course of a year, and his motivation no longer matched his vision.

His physical examination was significant for a somewhat more prominent fat layer, but otherwise unremarkable. His laboratory results demonstrated a number of decreased hormonal and nutrient factors that had potentially compromised his sense of well-being. Testosterone, dehydroepiandrosterone (DHEA), zinc, and thyroid hormone levels were all found to be suboptimal, and we addressed them appropriately in an effort to help him regain his focus and drive.

He recovered a great deal of his sense of well-being in the weeks that followed, leading to a significant increase in his ability to focus on his goals. He increased his efforts beyond those of his norm, and on his final follow-up, prior to competition, he related that he had created a space on his trophy wall for his upcoming win in the competition.

The infinite law of receiving is most simply understood as, "To give your best is to receive the best in ratio to the degree of your giving." It is another universal law that necessitates the accomplishment of more than one action in order to benefit fully from the law. It is critical to understand our place in the universal field of energy in order to exercise this law properly. This is the energy field that responds to our desires and beliefs and ultimately allows us to create whatever we desire in life. That creation is the practical result of applying the infinite laws to our lives. If the infinite law of supply has caused the creation of our desire for the thing we want, and our intention and expectation (law of attraction) help to draw us ever closer to this desired outcome, then the infinite law of receiving must define a condition of that receipt based upon the balance we have with the universal (quantum) energy of creation and supply.

This law, like all basic principles in the universe, is founded on the equilibrium we strike with our supplier of good. It is the dynamic parity required before any energy exchange can take place, whatever the form, and that includes our optimized health.

As Jesus said,

Give and it shall be given unto you: good measure, pressed down, shaken together, and running over will be put into thy bosom. For with the same measure that you use, it will be measured back to you. (Luke 6:38 NKJV)

If we see the equilibrium from an unbound perspective, one that allows us to look at receiving from the perspective of the recipient and the donor simultaneously, then receiving is giving, so we might read the passage as, "I have given, and it is given unto me." Since all material good is the result of creation from source (quantum) energy, it is only a matter of perspective. Also, the more we work with this energetic equilibrium, the more it works for us: "good measure, pressed down, shaken together, running over."

This is also true when we consider our health. We all want our health to be the best it can be. What is life without a healthy body to support it? For most of us, myself notwithstanding, when we consider something we desire, or anything in life for that matter, we often become focused on our understanding that we must receive of a thing before we can give of it. This displays our lack of understanding of how the law works. Therefore, to balance the energetic equilibrium, which cannot be maintained otherwise, we must initiate by giving before we may receive.

As expressed in Luke 6:38, in order to create from the energetic source of supply, the act of giving is fundamental before receiving can take place. So, if we continue to focus simply on "getting" good health, and our minds have this limited perspective, then it is unlikely we will achieve and receive the best health that we can have. I equate this attitude to thinking that we may achieve extraordinary health by taking a pill. Of course, that depends on perspective and how one defines extraordinary health and, of course, the abilities attributed to the pill. My own vision of extraordinary health is that of a happy child at play. I'm not at all certain we may accomplish that by taking a pill.

The law of receiving necessitates giving prior to getting, and as such, it is not unlike praying to receive a blessing. When we create a prayer, or in our case, as we create the mental image of our desired health, we create a vibration that is emitted from us to create (tether us to) our desired health. This is the quantum image we are imposing our belief upon. As this vibration is emitted outward to bind and to help us receive our desired supply, we then need to relax and prepare to receive the benefits from source. What this means is that our intent to achieve optimum health will transmit the vibration of expectation to our desired future in a quantum sense. Following this transmission, which is the giving factor, and depending upon the level of the vibration issued, we receive our desired improvements, or upgrades.

From a molecular biological perspective, what effect is this having on how the system is working? As previously discussed, our thoughts, beliefs, and actions of the past have generated our current health. Yes, it is time to own up; those thoughts and beliefs that we hold determine certain epigenetic expressions of our genes. Our expressions have manifested different beneficial and detrimental effects throughout our bodies and have created the result we have today. The efforts we take as we follow the guidance in this book are modifying those expressions, and will lead to our future selected healthy image.

There are an infinite number of health outcome possibilities, and an infinite number of time lines we can travel on to reach them. Any desired image we create may be achieved using our new talents and knowledge; that is the basis of these laws. Our thoughts and their vibrations systematically reach out and tether to our desired future health. Using the laws helps us keep the tether fixed, and then helps us to reel it in.

Many times I have heard patient-partners—even those in their thirties—say that they are too old to do something different. How can this even be a consideration for anyone? We learn to read when we are barely able to run across a schoolyard during the first five years of our lives. I might be a little more accepting of this attitude from a ninety-year-old whose health is compromised by multiple end-of-life organ failures. The truth is that we are capable of miraculous change and endeavors no matter what our age or physical condition. It is necessary only to create an image of what we want and it is ours. This is the law of supply, remember?

What does giving have to do with the law of receiving? Giving is, in part, in line with the imagined end results we send out with regard to our health. Our imagination creates excellent blood pressure, excellent blood sugar metabolism, excellent skeletal structure and function. And in our imagined intent we create a vibration of intensity similar to the level of desire for receipt. The vibration goes out and, if the environment (us) is prepared and ready, the supply (optimized health) will be received.

There may be a few small caveats to receiving that require clarification. When we do not perceive that we have the optimized health we want, we come from a position of lack or deprivation in our asking. Deprivation means that we previously had good health but no longer have it, and lack means we never had good health to begin with.

Lack and deprivation are disempowered states of being and are associated with the emotions of anger, craving, fear, anxiety, grief, regret, despair, guilt, and shame. These are very low vibrational energies and are typically associated with poor and/or declining health. Conversely, good health resides in the state of possession, which is an empowered state of being. The emotions associated with an empowered state of being include satisfaction, optimism, hopefulness, forgiveness, acceptance, love, serenity, joy, bliss, and enlightenment.

When we are imagining our optimized health, it is vital to do so from an empowered state of being. We cannot "ask" for optimized health from a space of lack or deprivation and expect to receive that which we are asking for. This is because, in the law of supply, that which we are "asking for" is already ours. Our optimized health is already ours! So, when we are presenting the "ask," what we ideally want to do is to express gratitude in advance—in faith, if you will—because that optimized health is already ours.

What is it that we must give in order to receive? Most people think of money as the substance of giving. Philosophically, money, by its very nature, is a form of energy obedient to our purposes, an agent of energetic exchange that discriminates only as far as we do. It is a symbol of the universal energy we have engaged by virtue of our desire to create, and it does our bidding as we see fit. If giving always precedes receiving, it is by virtue of our thoughts (which lead to action and/or belief), words (derived from your thoughts), actions and service (to yourself or others) that we serve the law and can commune with the positive results desired or intended.

In reality or practically, what does this mean and how does this affect our images in terms of achieving super man or super woman—ultimate health?

Let's think about this for a second. Giving of ourselves is the effort of preparing ourselves to receive the benefits of the improved health that we are asking for. Consider Roger's case. We are giving effort by virtue of our:

- **Thought**—This could mean, for example, thinking of new mental activities such as guided meditations, energy healing, and so forth, as well as new physical activities like low-impact exercising, yoga, tai chi, together with new spiritual activities. I am sure many of us have been advised to think of new ways to achieve our nutritional goals, like finding new recipes. Finally, our imaging activities—our mental effort or giving—are no less than thinking about our ultimate health outcome. This is attaching to supply. I refer back to the law of thinking, the basis of all your outcomes and conditions in life. Thought is a force of creation. It has the power to transform our health into the image we desire. It is how we communicate our health vision source, whereby it is created for us.

- **Words**—This means that your speech, by necessity, reflects only positive health affirmations. Only use positive affirmations in regards to your health, even if your mother always told you that you would be the sickly child.

  A fool's mouth is his destruction, and his lips are the snare of his soul. (Proverbs 18:7)
  A man's belly shall be satisfied with the fruit of his mouth; and with the increase of his lips shall he be filled. Death and life are in the power of the tongue; and they that love it shall eat the fruit thereof. (Proverbs 18:20, 21)

- **Actions**—This is characterized by decisive action on our exercise plans, nutritional plans, and mind-body exercises such as meditation, HeartMath training, and other disciplines.

  However many holy words you read, however many you speak, what good will they do you if you do not act upon them?

  —Buddha

- **Beliefs**—A belief is a personally assumed truth. It is not necessarily true or false, but is potentially beneficial, or even detrimental, particularly if the belief is based on incorrect information or assumption. In establishing beliefs, we must choose to seek out truthful, verifiable information to help ourselves as well as those around us. This means asking "why" and taking personal responsibility for finding the answers to our specific issues. It is of paramount importance that we confirm our information as correct, without assumption, as assumptions will give rise to incorrect beliefs that will be detrimental to our ultimate health outcome. Our beliefs set the stage for the most incredible potential outcomes that we can imagine—literally—for our health. It is the setting of belief that has quantum impact on our personal environment. Remember that the law of supply ultimately leads to the physical and bimolecular changes that determine our new health outcomes, and these can be whatever you wish them to be.

  Additionally, our subconscious minds do not have the ability to correct an erroneous notion. If we, say, I *can't*—fill in the blank—our subconscious minds will work to make sure that we can't. More importantly, if we say I *can*—fill in the same blank— I *am* … I *will* … I *have* … our subconscious minds will work on the appropriate responses to make those thoughts and beliefs come to fruition just as effectively. This is another reason to always believe you can. Your unfelt metabolism, through the conditioning of the subconscious, by the intermediary of your own genetic variability through epigenetic activation is driving the environment of your body to change for the better.

The next component of the law of receiving is preparing to receive. In preparing to receive, we display the active belief, or expectation, that we are going to have the anticipated response to our requests. Again, what we have imagined as a response or resolution to our health-related issue is what we will see in our future, by virtue of the law of supply. Now we need to prepare to receive. This also reinforces the law of thinking corollary that what we believe we will eventually see. We are also demonstrating faith and expectation as discussed in the law of attraction.

A fun example for those on weight-optimization programs is anticipatory shopping for new dresses or pants. Or, for those who are pursuing incremental physical conditioning, an example might be signing up for physical programs, on a future date, that require improved conditioning beyond that which you already have. These actions are signs of active faith and belief that our desired health image is ours. It keeps the image of success and intent vitalized and energizes the power of reception. It establishes the subconscious performance optimization to provide for the quantum input that generates the epigenetic changes that will lead to optimized healthy genetic expression.

You should also be wary of the converse situation, which may be the result of underlying limiting beliefs. Those beliefs are the ones that result in detrimental behavior or character traits. And for this, I bring you back to the teachings of Proverbs 12:14: "A man shall be satisfied with good by the fruit of his mouth" (KJV). And to the writing of Ms. Florence Shinn: "If one asks for success and prepares for failure, he will receive the situation he has prepared for."

Do not ask for success and prepare for the worst, or expect the worst. If you do, the worst is exactly what you will receive. The expectation of failure or, more simply, the feeling that you will not achieve success, will lead you to that end.

> *Argue for your limitations, and sure enough, they're yours.*
> —Richard Bach, author of *Jonathan Livingston Seagull*

Acts of preparing to receive also draw our heartfelt emotion and intent into play. They remove doubt, fear, misgivings, and other emotions that would impede reception or decrease the vibrational energy and thereby the strength of the tether that secures your attention to the expected image of success. Your expectations of good health increase, and success is based on the strength of your use of these simple and verified principles. You are the guide to the quality of the outcome by the attributes of your preparation. If the energy of receiving is a scalable quality, then the force and power of your preparation to receive great health by any action is then the key to your success.

Your Empowered Medicine Cabinet

An Addition to Your Morning Routine

What you want will come after you have first given of yourself.
—Dr. Trip Goolsby

In addition to continuing with the previous Medicine Cabinet processes, add this to your daily routine: Each morning as you prepare for your day, ask yourself this question: What is one new action I am committed to take today toward achieving my optimized health?

Maybe the answer is as simple as drinking more water and less alcohol, or taking the stairs as opposed to the elevator. Perhaps it is actually taking an experiential approach to the Empowered Medicine Cabinet processes, or finally signing up for a local marathon, or—dare I suggest—skipping Starbucks altogether?

Additionally, you are what you say you are, what you believe you are. So, develop some positive affirmations that are supportive of your personal ideal health image, and repeat them often. Here are some examples to get you started:

- I am vital and energetic.
- I am calm and relaxed grace.
- I am my optimal weight, and I maintain it.
- I am strong and flexible.
- I am of a healthy mind.

If this doesn't feel true for you in this moment, remember that it is with gratitude in faith that we form our affirmations as if we have already attained them, because, according to the law of supply, we already have.

CHAPTER 7

The Infinite Law of Increase in Health

I remember Christmas a few years back. I had not finished my shopping. This season is always somewhat stressful for me, and I cannot remember a season that has passed when Christmas Eve shopping was not on the list of things to do. The Christmas season I'm remembering was, however, punctuated by a new refrigerator magnet emblazoned with the following message to Santa Clause, "Dear Santa, I want it all! I want it now! And I want it delivered!" When I consider the condition and desires of most of my patient-partners upon initial evaluation, I often recall this quote. After all, we all want our recovered, optimized health right now, and we want it delivered, yes? This is where the law of increase comes into play.

The principle is to enhance, amplify, bolster, or accelerate the appearance of the results of our intended health image. Understanding this simple principle will assist you in resolving many chronic medical issues and keep your mind focused on those "happy end results."

Praise and gratitude are the avenues of enactment of this universal law. Accordingly, in my medical practice, a component of care requires the patient-partners to keep an ongoing gratitude journal. Consistently maintaining a gratitude journal serves up the practical aspect of being thankful and conditions us to think more profoundly into the true nature of our relationship with source. According to Raymond Holliwell, when we praise or thank God for the things we desire, "invariably the fulfillment of that desire is accelerated to almost magic proportion."

Praise and gratitude are of utmost importance. We are able to receive only those things (optimized health) for which we have a desire from the source of supply, accompanied by the belief and expectation of receipt. Remember, in that sense, asking or pleading is not an expectant posture. Recall our discussion of the vibrational energy of lack, which is not a vibrational match with the possession of optimized scintillating health. There is no sense of expectation when we panhandle for a moment of charity. Your expectant attitude is, therefore, one of affirmation, declaration, assertive thanksgiving, and gratitude of receipt—the claiming of the supply that has already been created for you. This means that your successful optimized health image is already yours, and you expedite your experience of it via grateful thanksgiving. Gratitude's character, defined by faith and expectancy, transmutes itself into the primary accelerant of the fire of universal benefit.

> *In Mark 11:24, Jesus says, "What things soever ye desire, when ye pray, believe*
> *that ye receive them and ye shall have them" (KJV).*

The law of increase stipulates that the expectant gratitude of having received the outcomes of our desires enhances the likelihood of receiving.

Not that praise or gratitude has any effect on Source. Source doesn't need our praise. Gratitude's effect has everything to do, however, with how our desired supply relates to us, and how it becomes available to us energetically. It is by lifting up our vibration energy level so that it matches that of our improved health—which is obviously at a higher energy level—that we are able to attain our improved health image. Gratitude and the feelings that accompany it are of a very high vibration energy and feeling. Gratitude places us and our conscious being on a higher plane of energy that allows us to grasp the desired health outcome and draw it to us.

> *The very disposition of the mind to gratitude, to glad acceptance, itself is power,*
> *carrying with it the gift to see and seize the best that*
> *every moment offers.*
> —James Allen, from comments on essays by M. Theobald

This concept of conscious energy elevation or vibration energy may need some clarification. David Hawkins, MD, PhD, actually correlated energy levels with different levels of consciousness and developed a scale of consciousness, which we will look at soon. The concept of vibrational levels of energy of all forms of matter and life was postulated in pre-antiquity by Egyptian philosophers around 5,000 BC. We are all made of atoms and elements and the biological substances that result from their combinations. Each atom and subatomic particle has an optimum frequency of vibration that defines the element. Likewise, different molecules and proteins have different vibrational frequencies that define their structures in the different phases of solid, liquid, and gas.

Water is, for example, the major component of your body, representing 60–65 percent of your total body weight. Water has specific measured vibrational frequencies depending on a number of variables including the physical state (solid, liquid, gas) and atomic bonding angles, and so forth. What that means is that we all have unique vibration frequencies based on our health, mood, ongoing levels of stress, activity, the ambient temperature, and on—and on, and on. Your emotional foundation and your ability to express gratitude are therefore simple means of achieving higher levels of vibratory energy without the need for boiling yourself!

Looking at the effect of simple mood and emotional exposures on water and how they affect its crystalline structure brings insight into the effects of the different emotions on the human being. Dr. Masaru Emoto analyzed the crystal structure of water that were exposed daily to love, hate, gratitude, and other emotions. The findings were astonishing in that the positive emotions elicited beautiful, organized, microscopic crystalline structures. The hateful, adversarial emotions caused the water to form into disorganized, chaotic structures. Thus, the positive feelings such as gratitude (which equate with love and appreciation) should attract much more positive outcomes than negative emotions, such as fear, guilt, shame, and anger. Imagine the protracted effects of positive affirmations about yourself in the setting of gratefulness, and then imagine the converse, if you are continually providing yourself with negative self-talk.

Because your vibrational energy is changing on a moment-to-moment basis, the energy levels documented in the scale of consciousness developed by Dr. David R. Hawkins and presented in his book, *Healing and Recovery*, provide you with a means by which you may try to alter your energy levels purposefully. Hawkins created the scale based on his tireless work with mindfulness and applied kinesiology.

The Map of Consciousness					
GOD-VIEW	LIFE-VIEW	LEVEL	LOG	EMOTION	PROCESS
Self	Is	Enlightenment	700-1000	Ineffable	Pure Consciousness
All-Being	Perfect	Peace	600 ↑	Bliss	Illumination
One	Complete	Joy	540 ↑	Serenity	Transfiguration
Loving	Benign	Love	500 ↑	Reverence	Revelation
Wise	Meaningful	Reason	400 ↑	Understanding	Abstraction
Merciful	Harmonious	Acceptance	350 ↑	Forgiveness	Transcendence
Inspiring	Hopeful	Willingness	310 ↑	Optimism	Intention
Enabling	Satisfactory	Neutrality	250 ↑	Trust	Release
Permitting	Feasible	Courage	200 ↑	Affirmation	Empowerment
Indifferent	Demanding	Pride	175 ↓	Scorn	Inflation
Vengeful	Antagonistic	Anger	150 ↓	Hate	Aggression
Denying	Disappointing	Desire	125 ↓	Craving	Enslavement
Punitive	Frightening	Fear	100 ↓	Anxiety	Withdrawal
Disdainful	Tragic	Grief	75 ↓	Regret	Despondency
Condemning	Hopeless	Apathy	50 ↓	Despair	Abdication
Vindictive	Evil	Guilt	30 ↓	Blame	Destruction
Despising	Miserable	Shame	20 ↓	Humiliation	Elimination

▓ The Final Doorway to Enlightenment/Nonduality
▓ The beginning of Integrity
▓ The beginning of the Nonlinear Realm

Notice the lower of the levels—the emotions of humiliation, blame, despair, regret, anxiety, craving, hate, and scorn. The use of motivational mindfulness modalities enables us to become more aware and attain higher, less-stressful vibrational levels. The higher the level we achieve, the more rapidly we will access and affirm the improved health image we desire.

Alternately, even the transmutation of a lower vibrational level of energy to a somewhat higher level progressively enables us to polish our subconscious goals to achieve progressively shinier results. This is simply the consequence of our vibrational frequencies reaching out to match those of progressively better results in well-being. In the act of being grateful for and praising the results we have already garnered, we have ever-improving results and can enhance the program we follow in a stepwise fashion.

Conversely, complaints, criticism, despair, and an anxious nature regarding the anticipated outcomes drive our vibration energy lower and delay or even disconnect us from our optimized health result. If we keep this in mind when we seem to reach the occasional plateau, we can recharge the batteries when we are grateful for the gains we have already achieved. It is important to plan a weekly reevaluation and assess the improvements and successes we have already accomplished. It is also important to be thankful for those recent past successes and, more importantly, for all those further improvements that will equally be ours.

Being grateful lifts our spirits, and the continued use of gratitude establishes transformational attitudes that draw in even further outcomes of greater benefit. Not unlike the way we are reminded to think on Thanksgiving Day, we should focus on the good that is in store for us, not just that which has already transpired. It is this belief in the health we have accomplished, and that is given to us in our image, that makes it come to pass. Believing leads to seeing! This is the faith that draws us to our tethered future outcome. By believing with gratitude in the image we have created, even when our current situation is full of challenges, whether multiple medical problems or results that seem to be awkwardly contrary, we enable our energy to remain high and fixed to our desired outcome.

We achieve what we expect and anticipate. We achieve what we believe and are grateful for. The active form of belief that enables us to express heartfelt gratitude and that raises our energy subsequently promotes a whole-body hormonal, metabolic, and immunologic transformational environment of healing and youthful regeneration. It activates positive epigenetic translational biomolecular pathways that endeavor to modify the foundations of our health.

It is in the setting of chronic diseases that the posture of the inverse paranoid—the person who chooses to believe that the world is plotting to do him or her good—is truly beneficial. It raises awareness to the motivational or transitional point of change, and in doing so, this grateful awareness and conscious optimistic perception transforms us in subtle ways that help to prevent further deterioration of well-being and health. The key to success in health is to shift perception of any setback or illness as a catalyst to achieve substantially better health in the near future.

I operate as though everyone is part of a plot
to enhance my well-being.
—Stan Dale, founder of the Human Awareness Institute

As we remain grateful and maintain affirmative expectation, our vibrational energy attracts better and better health. This is, in all likelihood, a foundational element in the successful Coué method of autosuggestion, which involved repeating the statement, "Every day, in every way, I'm getting better and better." This method, used successfully by Emile Coué, a French pharmacist and psychologist of the late nineteenth century, resulted in his patient population living with fewer illnesses and setbacks than patients of other physicians of the day.

Be ever grateful for the very least of things and the very
most will come to you.
—Raymond Holliwell

In this final quote, Holliwell reminds and summarizes for us that it is being grateful for the smallest of successes in our lives or lifestyle modification (even one pound of weight loss or one additional minute on the bike) that we reap the greatest long-term value in terms of the health related outcomes we can potentially attract.

Your Empowered Medicine Cabinet

Practice Gratitude

Your secret superpower is gratitude! In order to cultivate the habit of expressing gratitude in my family, every morning on the way to school, the kids and I each list ten things we are so thankful and grateful for. I do this because I understand that practicing conscious gratefulness opens the door for more of what I desire to come into my life.

The gratitude journal in the Appendix is your personal tool. Use it to begin cultivating your own habit of gratitude over the next two weeks. Each day, list at least ten things you are thankful for, and then take it one step further. Explain why you are thankful for the person, place, thing, and/or event. Really step into feeling your *why* when you do this, and repeat, "Thank you, thank you, thank you."

Within the two weeks, you will begin to notice subtle shifts in the ease and grace of your day. Your desire to engage in behavior that nourishes your body, yourself, and others will begin to take form. Consistency and authenticity are key as you begin to create this new habit of practicing conscious gratitude.

CHAPTER 8

The Infinite Law of Compensation in Health

Rita is a forty-nine-year-old, obese and diabetic woman who came in for evaluation of back pain, arthritis, hypertension, depression, anxiety, and mood instability. These issues had been repeatedly presented to her primary internist without significant evaluation or improvement. Despite the customary administration of sertraline and other selective serotonin reuptake inhibitors, the moodiness had worsened.

She had also noted significant increase in her weight along with worsening of her diabetes, which caused her to need more insulin. Her last menstrual period was approximately three years prior to her initial visit with me, but no hormone replacement therapy had been discussed or initiated. Her hypertension was controlled with prescription medications. Increasing back pain was her major complaint, and the pain was progressively limiting her daily activities. Rita used cigarettes to calm her anxiety and moodiness to the tune of fifteen to twenty cigarettes per day, a habit she had started when she was in her twenties. She had a scaly rash on both hands, and degenerative arthritic changes were visible on both hands. Imaging evaluations revealed a moderate reduction in bone density and some degenerative changes of the lumbar spine. Pulmonary function testing showed mild obstructive changes.

After initiating the appropriate hormonal replacement and nutritional and exercise lifestyle modifications, she began to feel significantly better. She was able to get off her antidepressant medications within three weeks after she began hormone replacement therapy. She quit smoking within six weeks without the use of medication. Now, after nine months, Rita has noted remarkable increase in her initiative and energy with no melancholic relapses.

More noticeable, perhaps, has been the transformative nature of her attitude of commitment and self-investment accompanying the mind-body behavioral modification training. Her new mood of excitement and forward thinking has completely obliterated that of her presenting persona, which dwelt consistently on the failures of the past and the dread of what possibly would befall her in the future.

Her diabetes was only a little more challenging. The delay in resolution was more the result of a few social hiccups, and giving rise to brief compliance related concerns, the total time necessary to eliminate her insulin therapy was about five months. At six and a half months, she no longer required prescription medications. Rita's weight is down substantially, and she continues to shrink. Her blood pressure, which is controlled with one medication, will succumb to her ongoing efforts shortly. Lastly, the arthritic complaints and bilateral rash are significantly improved, to the point of necessitating only occasional over-the-counter nonsteroidal anti-inflammatory medication. Rita's stress and resignation to the probability of having multiple complications from her diabetes and hypertension are now replaced by the energetic vision of a healthy future and a long, pain-free, fully functional and active life. Effort-related compensation? Let's see.

The law of compensation is another compound law. Setting the stage for this most important of laws—particularly insofar as concerns the acquisition of health and well-being—is the concept of universal wholeness, the completion of what, at first blush, would seem to be competing polarities.

> *An inevitable dualism bisects nature so that each thing is half and suggests another thing to make it whole; as, spirit, matter; man, woman; odd, even; subjective, objective; in, out; upper, under; motion, rest; yea, nay. While the world is thus dual, so is every one of its parts.*
> —Ralph Waldo Emerson, *Essays: First Series: Compensation* (1841)

The respective polarities are a part of a continuum that reveals itself only as dependent on the perspective of the viewer. In his essays, Emerson also wrote,

> *There is always some leveling circumstance that puts down the overbearing, the strong, the rich, the fortunate, substantially on the same ground with all others. Is a man too strong and fierce for society and by temper and disposition a bad citizen … nature sends him a troop of pretty sons and daughters, who are getting along in the dame's classes at the village school, and love and fear for them smooths his grim scowl to courtesy.*

This universal law compels us to recognize the balance that is due in every sector of life, including our health. It is in this sense that our efforts of creating a new biologic and hormonal balance, revitalizing our mind-body optimization, rejuvenating our physical activity as well as initiating robust nutritional and nutraceutical optimization will bourgeon into the positive health benefits that we have conceived. When we consider what we are doing from a biomolecular perspective, we will be compensated for our efforts of optimization by improved epigenetic performance within our bodies over time. Remember, the cellular turnover in our bodies is complete within seven years.

The law helps those who help themselves. Or, more simply, your efforts will be compensated to whatever degree you give or contribute. This is the most basic representation of the law as it is currently stated. It is a law requiring and imposing a force of action and strength to the participants. In fact, this is not at all dissimilar from the law of karma: we will reap what we sow. The Bible teaches the same:

"Whatsoever a man sows, that shall he also reap" (Galatians 6:7 KJV).

We, and our health, are the prisoners of the thoughts and beliefs we hold closest.

Understanding their impact and how we may use them is the key to our optimized health freedom—the key to freeing ourselves from the burdens of poor health. We are, most of us, compromised by the baggage of detrimental beliefs we developed over the years. These limiting beliefs, created by the trust we placed in our intimate advisors for our health (parents, physicians, friends, pharmacists, colleagues, acquaintances, and pseudoscientific Internet resources) are amplified and ingrained by repetition, and we now reap the health benefits we have sown by compounding the confusion of the lessons of "trusted" advisors, inadvertently or not. We are being compensated, like it or not. This is the health karma that we are generating for ourselves and spreading to those around us.

Our health is a reflection of our ruling thoughts, as well as the prevailing vision of our health. The mind, the limiting beliefs, and their resultant manifestations, with few exceptions, are the sites that require intervention. *Health is the impact of reflection and action of knowledgeable belief manifestations.* If we believe we are healthy and will remain so, and our beliefs are founded in right thoughts, actions, and habits, then we will truly remain healthy and vibrant for years. The classic examples of this are Jack LaLanne and other perceived mentors of health and fitness over the years. Those who have exemplified protracted health believe in maintaining optimized metabolic and hormonal balance, nutrition, exercise, mindbody coherence, alongside an optimized vision of future health that is focused on attracting well-being in lieu of disease. Yes, this means your verbalizations of negative health outcomes must cease yesterday!

We must consistently and deliberately make only positive statements about our health, even if in the moment it may not appear or feel "real." At all costs, refrain from speaking any statements like these:

- I'm always sick.
- I always get the flu.
- I'm going to get cancer.
- My family has diabetes, so I'm sure I'm going to get it.

Statements like these only serve to set the stage for the acquisition of negative results by placing us on the same energy level of the ailments and diseases. These statements are verbal invitations. We simply open the door and let them in.

Remember, our supply is ever present, and anything we ask for, any demands we place on the ethereal, quantum supply will be provided. This will happen, regardless of what we might think is a simple frivolous jest.

> *Accidents, old age, and death itself come from holding wrong mental pictures.*
> *When a man sees himself as God sees him, he will become a radiant being,*
> *timeless, birth-less, and deathless.*
> —Florence Shinn, author of *Your Word Is Your Wand* (1928)

The good news is that the law will always work, and our active effort to change our thoughts, actions, and beliefs related to our health will achieve these results for us over time. The changes we reap will be the compensation for the effort we apply. Think about the result of the bodybuilder who uses progressively heavier and heavier weights and continues with the exercises. The neuro-connectivity for that thought will grow stronger and stronger over time.

There are no bargains to be had in this domain, however. The law of compensation is complementary to the law of cause and effect. It produces according to its rule of action. If we are healthy, happy, and wealthy, then we are being compensated according to our actions. The converse is also true. So, in understanding this and the previous laws, we move forward to procure our health with the understanding that it is possible to have any health we want from any starting point we have. All things are possible, starting with our first thought, our first image. They are the investments from which we will receive compensation over and over and over again.

We must become more aware of how we perceive our choices and make decisions regarding our health-related actions. Conscious decisions may, at some times, be more difficult than at other times. Our heartfelt intuition and intuitive sensory responses can oftentimes supplant the need for laborious research and contemplation in the heat of the moment. These "gut-level" responses are connected with infinite intelligence and may serve as a guide to spontaneous health-related decision making. Intuitive impressions may be obtained by any number of methods, including muscle testing, gut feelings, among others. A positive intuitive response is generally accompanied by a positive sense of well-being, a sense of relaxed reassurance. If the action being contemplated will be of nefarious health value, the sensation will be ominous, and the action should be avoided. We need to be aware of subconscious decisions that take place in an almost reflex fashion, and that may contribute to adversely impacting the epigenetic manifestations of our cells. Awareness in the moment of our health-related decisions is the only way we accomplish this feat, and it will be a significant promulgator of well-being in our lives.

If we are looking for the good in ourselves, as opposed to engaging in self-criticism and negative self-talk, then we are able to evolve into individuals who truly love, nurture, and honor ourselves. This will then naturally begin to reveal itself in the status of our health and overall quality of life. This is critical in respect to our optimized health for two reasons:

1. We will continually be focused on our optimum outcome and health perfection as we see it in the moment.
2. The focus on condemnation or a negative judgment of a health status or outcome creates an environment of stress within our bodies—subconsciously if not consciously—with its resulting adverse hormonal and metabolic environment.

> *Turn the energy of your mind upon ideas of plenty, love, happiness, joy, health*
> *and they, in turn, will appear.*
>
> —Raymond Holliwell

Compensation is also defined as a reward or an appropriate benefit in exchange for a service, a loss, a debt, or a defect. In biological terms, or in terms of our well-being, this would mean the development of improved (compensatory) function in a different area of the same organ that had a functional deficit, or compensatory improvement in an ability in order to make up for a defective organ function. We see this happen frequently in the development of acquired nervous system defects, as in stroke recovery, for example, or improved hearing in those who lose their sight. Psychologically the use of a substitutive behavior to make up for a deficient, or perceived deficient, behavior has also been frequently noted.

If we want better health, the law of compensation would have us sow the idea of, and prepare for, better health by focusing the energy of our thought on the desired outcome. To do this we must be thankful and grateful for whatever health foundation we have, as this is the springboard from which we will bound to the next level.

> *Success requires no explanations; failure allows no alibis.*
> —Napoleon Hill, author of *Think and Grow Rich*

Many of our successes, as convalescents, are derived by the law of compensation and the law of receiving, most certainly for those recovering from adult onset diabetes and obesity. The most profound results are obtained when our patients more fully engage the use of the imaging and autosuggestion exercises (positive affirmations). These are enhanced by association with the brainwave entrainment programming we recommend. I recommend their daily use both morning and evening, and at times of heightened stress that threaten failure or noncompliance. Another reason for failure, which is more subtly related to noncompliance with the law of compensation, is expecting something for nothing or expecting a fabulous outcome for a perceived bargain. How can we expect to improve upon our condition while contributing little or nothing to the effort?

Let's not dwell at length here on the promises of pharmaceuticals that currently base their results on the law of averages, so to speak: positive medical effects, for some, balanced with adverse side effects for an "acceptable" portion of users. Each of us has a different constitutional makeup (read: genome) and our individual health situations require individual approaches for optimum outcomes. This is the premise of precision medicine that is being researched and applied using the results of the Human Genome Project and epigenomic medicine.

That said, this misconception of ideal results without compensatory effort based on the use of a pharmaceutical is a difficult one to unsell from the mind of the patient and the physician. I can no longer count the number of long-term complicated diabetics that I have been able to take off insulin therapy and oral medication. The simple use of lifestyle modification and hormone optimization results in complete resolution of their "disease." Need I discuss hypertensive patients and depression? We are, patients and physicians alike, reaping what we have sown.

We contribute nothing to be compensated for when we do not give our time, service, and effort to inform ourselves and surround ourselves with the people, providers, and information necessary to make the decisions that will garner the health success we deserve.

Your Empowered Medicine Cabinet

Energy In = Energy Out!

There is no doubt that you have been diligently applying the "medicine" from the previous chapters, and are also mindfully and successfully working through your gratitude journal. Keep it up!

Here, we are going to consider the practical application of the law of compensation in health. Again, this law, simply stated, is that the degree of the input will equal the degree of the output. Energy in equals energy out.

For some reason, this concept is really easy for us to understand and apply as it relates to our careers and jobs: Do the work, get paid. Don't do the work, don't get paid, or worse, get fired. Yet we space out on this law when it comes to almost anything else, such as our relationships or our health.

You picked up this book because something about it resonated with you—the title, *Empowered Medicine*, the picture. Perhaps it was the table of contents. Whatever it was, your attraction to the book means that there is an aspect of you that is ready for an improved health status. There is an aspect of you that already recognizes that the effort you have been putting into your health is insufficient to achieve the change you truly desire. So, you bought this book, and now you are actually reading it and applying the laws and using them as an experiential tool. Congratulations! You are engaging in the law of compensation, and with consistent, mindful application, you will begin to see the results of your efforts. It can be no other way: energy in = energy out.

Ask yourself the following:

- What do I want with respect to my optimized health? (Revisit the "Visualize Your Health" Medicine Cabinet at the end of Chapter 2 and brush up on and optimize your successful health image via the Form, Feeling, and Function process and handout.)
- Why do I want it? (What awesome and amazing things will I do? What grand places will I travel to? How energetic, vibrant, and alive will I finally feel?)
- And how much effort (energy), am I willing to put into getting it?

CHAPTER 9

The Infinite Law of Allowance in Health

This is a law we need to use correctly on a daily basis. Using it not only gives significant perspective on what our optimum health might be, but also provides us with a resource for peace and relief of stress. This latter benefit is extremely useful in the prevention and reduction of certain disease processes. Hypertension and diabetes are primary examples.

Today I must have discussed the basics of allowance with at least five patients. "I'm still struggling to lose the weight I want to lose." "I'm fighting my cancer." "I'm going to beat this depression and anxiety." This is the daily chorus that greets me as I reach into the universal energy and provide what I hope is some small clarification on the use of the law of nonresistance to the patients who are not quite yet attuned to the guidance that is being provided to them by these disease processes.

When we reflect more deeply about the equilibrium necessary for creativity in terms of our health, we understand that harmony and synchronicity with the universal laws enables us to best obtain our empowered health ideal. That is to say, when we relax into harmonious alignment, when we step into allowance, that is when we open the doors to that which we desire to come through. So, if it is good health we desire, then our thoughts, beliefs, actions, and routine habits must be aligned with our desires.

Here is the easiest way to state this law: ***What we resist persists.*** With everything in life, particularly our health, whatever we struggle to remedy, whatever we brace for with our steeled willpower cannot be resolved because our consistent resistance perpetuates consistent persistence. How can this be so?

The infinite laws are uniformly based on harmony and equilibrium, so is it possible to create balance and equilibrium by answering the call of the annoyance with a resistant response? Two objects colliding at whatever speed, with whatever momentum do not make for a pretty outcome in most cases. This is comparable to the irresistible force paradox, which asks what happens when an unstoppable force meets an immovable object. Insofar as concerns our health, is it possible, for example, to decrease the stress on an organ system by creating an opposing stress? No.

Let's think about diabetes for a minute. An elevated blood sugar level is, in most cases, the result of inadequate insulin or inadequate activity of insulin due to quantity or quality (ability to be active). Now let's add the idea of resistance to this disease state. Resistance, of whatever type, would be considered a new stress because it is an opposing force to the acquisition of harmony and equilibrium. What does that yield in the context of our bodies and health? Stress of any sort activates a *stress response*. And this response in our bodies creates a reactive environment with even more adverse biochemical and hormonal conditions that prevent insulin from doing its job. From the metabolic and hormonal perspective, the presence of the increased concentrations of cortisol, epinephrine, and growth and hormones during a stress response, requires significantly higher concentrations of insulin in order for insulin to accomplish its role. *Fighting* diabetes creates a stress response, which leads to greater disequilibrium and disease aggravation.

The infinite law of allowance requires that we ***focus our energy on our successful health while accepting our current status***. By accepting and taking responsibility for our current health, we raise our vibrational energy to harmonize with the improved health we desire. We are no longer fighting, blaming, or resisting our current undesired health status. There is a proverb in which a man tells a friend he feels as if he has two fighting wolves inside him, an evil wolf and a good wolf. "Which one wins?" his friend asks. "The one I feed," the man replies. So, we feed the wrong wolf with any time or effort we expend on thoughts, complaints, or discussions of what we *don't* want (obesity, pain, fatigue, lack of energy, and so forth). As we focus our energy in the "fight" against our health situation, we deplete our resources. We are better served when we center our attention on the positive energy that is associated with harmonizing with that image we have already set as our optimized health.

Our focus must be, at all times, on those attributes that we want and expect to have. This is the law of supply and the law of attraction at work. Any obstacle that we may face as we move toward achieving our optimum health is the result of our past thoughts, actions, and beliefs. In this acknowledgment we become nonresistant to the challenge or situation, and thus create the momentum for innovative improvements. This moment of release will be, in most instances, followed by intuitive ideas and what we perceive to be epiphanies that assist in constructive, positive resolution. Knowing and accepting our health as it exists flows with the universal harmony that is and allows universal knowledge and resources to flow to us for creative inspiration and assistance.

Whatever we do, we need not worry about the potential solution or the existing challenge. I'll say it again: ***worry represents resistance***. The sense of relaxation and comfort will accompany the release experience. We are no longer choosing to create stress in our bodies, and instead are creating a healthier metabolic and immune environment in our bodies.

How do we achieve the ideal health we are imaging with our exercises? By accepting ourselves and our health as it is right now, no exceptions. It is what it is. When we are grateful for our awareness, which allows us to conceptualize our current health status and the information it provides, that acknowledgment places us directly into the state of allowance.

I often use a metaphor of a small stream as it grows to become a river. The stream frequently changes its route along the way to becoming a river. Think about the Mississippi at its origins. The small stream is not strong enough to displace even the smallest obstacle, so it circumnavigates many of them. As it gains power and strength, it is finally capable of displacing some obstacles. Not only does this action continue to move the stream closer to its larger, more forceful self, it often gives it perspective to better pathways to take along the way. Slowing to fight a larger stone or stem, rather than flowing around it, creates energetic waste.

Simply allowing any setbacks and challenges as they may arise is part of the path to our optimized health status. Consider obstacles and challenges as opportunities, perhaps even as blessings because they may, even if we are not aware at the moment, present shortcuts or detours that could take us closer to our health goals. Liken it to being treated to an incredible view of fall foliage that you would have missed it hadn't been for an "annoying" detour you had to take when an accident blocked the road. Bless the obstacle and move on!

With this new perspective on our health, we are now able to demonstrate acceptance of the health we currently possess. With this new understanding, the situation becomes the fault of no single individual or event; neither are we at fault for its creation. We know that this is the universe at work in our favor, and all is as it should be. From this new perspective, we have the opportunity to choose to respond in peace, harmony, creativity, and decisiveness.

Finally, this response of allowance provides us with the demeanor of gratitude and the elevated vibrational energy of joy that accompanies it, facilitating the acquisition of improved health. And so, like the stream growing into the river, the momentum of an empowered health outcome grows!

Your Empowered Medicine Cabinet

Learn the Benefit of Allowing

This is probably one of the most difficult universal laws for many people to apply. The concept is simple enough, but it is somewhat counterintuitive, right?

Think back to that scene in the first Harry Potter movie, *The Sorcerer's Stone* (2001), in which Harry, Ron, and Hermoine struggle against devil's snare. Hermoine tells Harry and Ron, "Stop moving, both of you. This is devil's snare! You have to relax. If you don't, it will only kill you faster!"

This is the perfect example of being in resistance to that which we do not want. It is the opposite of allowance. Resistance blocks what we want. In Harry, Ron, and Hermoine's case, they want to live!

Chinese handcuffs are also another great example of the importance of allowance. As you try to get your fingers out of the woven cylinder, the more you struggle and pull, the tighter the hold of the handcuffs.

So, how do we get into a space of allowance? By first realizing that we are in a space of resistance. If we are "fighting," "struggling," "pushing against," if we feel as if we have to go upstream, notice this: if all of our efforts appear to be generating more and more of whatever we no longer desire (compromised health), perhaps it is time to make a different choice. Maybe it is time to relax into allowance. It's just a conscious choice on our part to release all that struggle because it is just no longer serving us.

There are several great mantras to use when relaxing into allowance seems to be counterintuitive. The first one is "All is well." I sometimes like to say, "Nothing I want is upstream." I frequently repeat these over and over again until I believe them, and then my reality begins to "see" them.

Give it a try and let me know how it works for you.

CHAPTER 10

The Infinite Law of Forgiveness in Health

Remember Steven, the forty-two-year-old smoker from chapter 5—The Infinite Law of Attraction in Health? In addition to his other chronic health issues, Steven presented with a one-to one-and-a-half-pack-per-day smoking habit. However, within a short period of time after coming to see me, Steven began to respond quite well to the smoking cessation process I use in my practice.

This process involves what we call "The Why List." First, the patient-partner must make a list of what circumstances make him or her want to smoke the cigarettes. I call this the "triggering why" list. Second, the patient-partner must determine why in the world he or she is wishing to smoke a cigarette in the first place. I call this the "philosophical why." This second part involves writing down a potentially negative outcome from smoking, which always includes conditions such as cancer, COPD, heart attack, strokes, and so forth. Third and last, the patient-partner must choose an activity to replace the act of smoking for each different "triggering why." This "replacement list" might include such things as chewing gum, sucking on candy, biting fingernails, chewing on a pen cap, running a mile or two, and so on. Vaping is not permitted as a replacement activity.

After completing these exercises, the patient-partner sets a date for cessation. The plan, for the most part, is for the patient-partner to taper consumption significantly by enacting the suggestions on the "replacement list." Total cessation is then easily achieved. This is, in part, a practical application of the Infinite Law of Forgiveness in Health, as you will see.

The knowledge base that has been provided by the Human Genome Project and ongoing research into various epigenetic modulations enables us to create precision programs for individuals. These programs take into account the risk and individual genomic responses to different lifetime exposures.

The diseases that place the largest burden upon us are those brought about by our own errant behavior. The thoughts that stem from erroneous beliefs and that lead to the behaviors that do not serve our optimized health status are often the origin of aggravating diseases. Once these errant behaviors are recognized and acknowledged, they must then be forgiven. This may sound a bit cryptic, so I will endeavor to clarify.

Let's consider our bodies and how they acquire disease: it is by virtue of our exposures. Our bodies are a result of the manifestations of our inherited genetic material. Our exposures may be acquired from outside our bodies in the form of bacteria, viruses, fungi, parasites of diverse sorts, toxins of a chemical or physical nature, and so forth. But exposures can also come from inside, and these are mostly mental in origin. The effects of these exposures, or insults, may manifest immediately. Examples are infections and acute trauma, among others. They may also manifest over the long term by affecting our genetic material. There is a delay in the appearance of symptoms, and the length of the delay is based on the reserve of the individual and the organ system(s) involved.

The body is similar to a petri dish, those small dishes that scientists use to culture everything from bacteria to sheep and individual body parts. Scientists place whatever cell type they want into whatever solutions they deem necessary to obtain the desired end result. Our bodies are very much like those petri dishes in that we expose the entire cellular content to different culture mediums, beneficial or not, throughout the day every day, and throughout our lives via the circulating blood. The content of the fluids that our cells are exposed to, insulting or not, determines how the cells express the genes we are given by our parents.

A disease is the result of the distribution, through the solution of the petri dish, of insulting substances (toxicities) or other agents of harm. The subsequent physical manifestations that are brought about by the insults follow patterns that are well documented, in most cases, and can be more or less disagreeable, even fatal. (Sounds like a pharmaceutical commercial, doesn't it?) The toxic exposures we incur come to us from the outside environment or result from stressors that we create ourselves through the process of thinking. In most cases, multiple simultaneous or sequential attacks are responsible for the ensuing disease.

> *I have had many worries in my life, some of them were even real.*
>
> —Mark Twain

Aditi Nerurkar, MD, MPH; Asaf Bitton, MD, MPH; Roger B. Davis, ScD; et al, wrote an article entitled "When Physicians Counsel About Stress: Results of a National Study" (*Journal of the American Medical Association, Internal Medicine* 2013;173[1]:76–77). Their study found that 60–80 percent of all primary care visits are related to stress. It seems that an internal cause of disease should be considered the most prevalent. And, following my petri dish analogy, we may conclude that the thoughts of an individual, which create the internal environment of the body, are the major contributors to ill health.

Multiple clinical and inferential epidemiological studies have documented the nefarious effects of stress on the onset and/or worsening of psychiatric disease. But cardiovascular disease, immunological effectiveness and malfunction, along with the outcomes of many different individual diseases may be affected as well. These statements have likewise been corroborated in the *Journal of the American Medical Association* article entitled, "Psychological Stress and Disease" in which psychologists at Carnegie Melon University reviewed and noted the contributions of stress to multiple diseases, both psychiatric and nonpsychiatric. Evidence in at-risk populations show significant increases in the incidence, progression, and adverse outcomes of cardiovascular disease, autoimmune disease, HIV, cancer, upper respiratory tract infections, herpes viral infections, and wound healing deficiencies.

We must take stock of the number of ideas and beliefs we hold, either consciously or subconsciously, that may be actively impairing our perfect health and our ability to achieve it. Antiquated past beliefs or perceived knowledge that we continually focus on, either consciously or subconsciously, must be eliminated in order to empower an updated, reinforced healthy image for the future. How is this accomplished? We do it by forgiving that thought or belief that limits our empowered image of exuberant well-being. We may have more difficulty clearing these ideas and beliefs if they are longstanding and have been implanted by others that we trust or have trusted even in the recent past. I refer here to limiting beliefs that may be imparted by health care practitioners unfamiliar with the improved outcomes obtained with optimized integrated modalities.

The idea of forgiveness here refers to eliminating the originating (erroneous) thought or idea that was installed. We do this by forgiving, which means forsaking and forgetting it. That same forgiveness is, in effect, the replacement of erroneous information by good information. Unless we can eliminate these limiting ideas—bad information—from our conscious and subconscious thoughts, we will not be capable of implanting or implementing new invigorating, constructive, healthy ones.

Solomon relates in Proverbs 28:13, "He that covers his sins [limiting beliefs, ideas, thoughts] shall not prosper: but whoever confesses [recognizes] and forsakes [corrects] them shall have mercy [be forgiven]" (AKJV).

Keep in mind that this and numerous additional verses in the Bible equate thought with sin and vice versa. So any erroneous thought may be considered the equal of a sin. And subsequently, Raymond Holliwell, in *Working with the Law: 11 Truth Principles for Successful Living*, said, "A sin forsaken is a sin forgiven."

In *Byways of Blessedness,* James Allen reflected on forgiveness:

> *The hard-hearted and unforgiving suffer most … for not only do they, by the law of attraction, draw to themselves the revengeful passions in other people, but their hardness of heart itself is a continual source of suffering. Every time a man hardens his heart against a fellow being, he inflicts upon himself five kinds of suffering—namely, the suffering of loss of love; the suffering of the loss of communion and fellowship; the suffering of a troubled and confused mind; the suffering of wounded passion or pride; and the suffering of punishment inflicted by others … whereas the act of forgiveness brings the doer five kinds of blessedness—the blessedness of love; the blessedness of increased communion and fellowship; the blessedness of a calm and peaceful mind; the blessedness of passion stilled and pride overcome; and the blessedness of kindness and goodwill bestowed by others.*

When we forgive, we are forgetting, abandoning, correcting, and relinquishing the condition (disease), thoughts (wrong ideas and concepts) or persons who prompted the enactment of the wrongdoing, insult, or offense that has taken place. We are replacing bad information with good. The act of forgiveness enables us to create a higher vibrational energy of prosperity, health, happiness, and abundance. It does so by eliminating the adversarial low-energy thoughts that take us to a lower energy consciousness. Read again: bad information will result in adverse outcomes that will create stress, malaise, disease, and therefore a low-energy consciousness that is self-perpetuating. Forgiving enables us to move forward to an invigorating, energetic, and healthy life!

When we reflect further on the wrongdoing, we invariably realize that we are living in the past or, by virtue of our imaginations, the hypothetical future. These fictional, imaginary disenfranchising scenarios prevent us from focusing on the positive elements of our future goals for optimized health. We are delivering our reserves of energy and strength to the thing that has created stress and misgivings within our lives. The stress response then goes on and on, aggravating the metabolic and endocrine imbroglio that worsens inflammation, blood pressure, diabetes, insomnia, as well as creating more difficulties with memory, attitude, anxiety, depression, irritability, pain, fatigue, and chronic illness. I often use the analogy of "driving in the rearview mirror." This activity is one that also invariably leads to collisions of unimaginable magnitude with more blocks and obvious painful outcomes.

In my practice we use focused imaging, which creates an empowering and ideal health image. For many, we also use biofeedback, which reinforces forgiveness, and centers conscious and subconscious thoughts on valid affirmative goals for optimized health. It is when the physician/practitioner who is involved in the patient-partner relationship becomes the partner-coach/counselor/teacher that he or she truly becomes the agent that promotes forgiveness.

Your Empowered Medicine Cabinet

Make Your Lists

Here we are going to implement the "Why List" and the "Replacement List" as explained in the preceding chapter. While this process is most often used for our smoking cessation program, it is possible to use for any addiction or negative behavior that you desire to overcome, such as overeating. The steps again are as follows:

(1) The Triggering Why:

Write down your answer or answers to the following questions:

- What is my why?
- Why am I choosing to engage in [fill in the blank]?
- What are my triggers?

(2) The Philosophical Why:

Write down your answer or answers to the following question:

Why in the world am I wishing to [fill in the blank] in the first place?

This step involves writing down a potentially disempowering outcome from your [fill in the blank]. Examples could be cancer, COPD, heart attack, strokes, and so forth.

(3) The Replacement List:

Finally, you must determine an activity to replace the act of your [fill in the blank] Examples could be chewing gum, sucking on candy, biting fingernails, chewing on a pen cap, running a mile or two, and so forth.

Do this step for each for each different "triggering why."

After completing this process, set a goal date for no longer engaging in the addiction/ behavior. Write it down and post it up somewhere where you will see it every day. You can do it!

CHAPTER 11

The Infinite Law of Sacrifice in Health

Jane is a forty-two-year-young vibrant woman with a history of malignant melanoma. She came to see me for evaluation of multiple problems related to obesity, weight gain, and moodiness with persistent fatigue, easy fatigability, and poor tolerance of her oral antidepressants. One of her greatest desires, along with resolution of the presenting complaints, was to achieve a bikini body by the upcoming summer beach season.

She had undergone a total hysterectomy in her late thirties without hormone replacement. She was placed on antidepressant therapy approximately six months following her hysterectomy. Significant weight gain accumulated shortly thereafter. Her only other historical therapeutic intervention was chemotherapy, which she received following her surgery for malignant melanoma. Her thyroid function was found to be suboptimal during my evaluation, and required attention.

As part of my initial evaluation of my patient-partners, I have them record a two-week nutritional diary. I use this to assess the nature of their alimentary intake. Jane's nutritional diary was similar to that of most inhabitants of southern Louisiana. This included lots of rice, bread, gravy, gumbo, and *boudin* (a type of Cajun sausage). Jane's beverage of choice was Dr Pepper, and she consumed three to six cans per day.

Following completion of her evaluations, I instituted hormonal optimization. This included using replacement bioidentical estradiol, progesterone, and testosterone, as well as addressing her suboptimal thyroid function with Armour thyroid. I had my customary nutritional discussion with her, focusing on the elimination of a large part of the carbohydrate load that she was consuming. Finally, we discussed an exercise regimen, as well as her initiation of our proprietary mind-body program.

Jane initially responded quite well to the hormonal and nutritional modifications, and we were soon able to taper off and discontinue her antidepressant. However, she stagnated rapidly in her fitness acquisition, despite assuring me that she was following the nutritional and exercise guidelines that we established together. Her follow-up laboratory evaluations were, in fact, significantly improved from her initial ones, but her A1C test showed her average blood glucose levels were still high. I asked her to keep another two-week nutrition diary. Two weeks later when she returned, I found the she was continuing to pursue multiple Dr Pepper consultations daily. I indicated that it might be necessary to seek the opinions of an alternative specialty that would be more considerate of her goals, particularly the bikini season physique. Pursuing the sacrifice of multiple daily Dr Pepper consultations, Jane subsequently found her weight loss groove again, and her glycemic control was enhanced to acquire a normalized A1C.

The infinite law of sacrifice in health has very different meanings and implications for everyone. The truth of the matter, however, is that for everything we wish to achieve or do achieve, we must sacrifice something (or something is sacrificed) in return for the accomplishment. The law states that to obtain something we desire, something must always be sacrificed. These sacrifices are never casual in nature, but the sacrifice is generally made in anticipation of the reception of a greater good. Our empowered health corollary is, by necessity, that we must anticipate that, **for each advance or improvement in health, we must choose to sacrifice a less-desirable health character and/or habit.**

It would seem that this law is quite complimentary to the laws of receiving and compensation, and it is. The main issue is that we must anticipate the sacrifice with the discipline necessary to make it happen. By forfeiting or sacrificing a habit, we then receive (are compensated with) what we truly desire in the long term. It is healthier to forfeit the characteristic or habit that we intuitively perceive needs to go than it is to have something unexpected befall us as the result of undisciplined or ignorant self-neglect. This self-neglect may be true from many perspectives as we live our lives and consume our extraordinary reserve.

Each of the different organ systems responds to different beneficial and compromising inputs from our interior and exterior environments. The inputs activate the epigenetic cascade in an affirmative or adversarial fashion, finally yielding consumption, enhancement, or no change in the reserve we possess.

In Matthew 7:14, Jesus relates, "Straight is the gate, and narrow is the way, which leadeth unto life, and few there be that find it" (KJV).

From a health perspective, the infinite law of sacrifice could be translated thus: the wealth of life that is available for us is abundant. But it is not by virtue of simple chance or a serendipitous lifestyle ignorant of healthy behavior that we will achieve it. A disciplined informed lifestyle is necessary to achieve our desired goals and the abundant empowered life for each individual—whatever that may be.

> *It is one of the paradoxes of Truth that we gain by giving up; we lose by greedily grasping. Every gain in virtue necessitates some loss in vice; every accession of holiness means some selfish pleasure yielded up; and every forward step on the path of Truth demands the forfeit of some self-assertive error.*

> —James Allen

The discipline we all must seek in the setting of acquiring our optimized health is much more often related to this sacrifice and loss in order to gain and advance in our physical and mental well-being. Conversely, there is an absence of discipline to eliminate the undesirable behavior (the ones that are likely contributing to the progression and maintenance of undesirable epigenetic activity). This is exemplified, for example, by the consumption of carbohydrates in the setting of type 2 diabetes, or cigarette smoking in the setting of chronic bronchitis, and is clearly disobedient to the law garnering its own anticipated outcome.

Those elements in our lives that are beneficial and serve us are generally not the ones that will need to be eliminated (sacrificed), obviously. Those that are detrimental by virtue of their unconscious and/or uninformed nature will need to be sacrificed to the benefit of our health. Additionally, the investment we release (the sacrifice made) and the effort of our giving (infinite law of receiving) create a superior value for the empowered outcome we desire. These two infinite laws then become the currency by which we determine the health compensation for the health outcome we envision. Insofar as it holds true for our empowered health optimization, we need not sacrifice for optimization in the areas that are clearly good; we need only sacrifice the bad and discipline ourselves in those areas that are painful and hinder our optimum health. Should we acquire any significant health advantage without providing the necessary sacrifice (personal investment), it is unlikely we will truly perceive any long-term benefit.

An easy health and wellness example of this concept is trying to lose weight with the use of pharmaceuticals or through a surgical procedure. These pathways to weight loss are often fraught with a high degree of failure by the simple fact that there is little or no value attributed to the achievement. A recent long-term follow-up study of laparoscopic surgical banding of the stomach revealed a high overall failure rate. Other studies corroborated this fact by finding greater than 25 percent of failure within eighteen months and only 40 percent long-term weight loss success (in other words, 60 percent failure at ten years) with this popular procedure. Oral weight loss medications are routinely known to have a high incidence of rebound obesity and are complicated often by hypertension and long-term damage to the heart.

Another interesting example here would be our suboptimal nutritional lifestyle. For the most part we should sacrifice (avoid) high-glycemic-index carbohydrate loads (foods that make our blood sugar levels rise rapidly). High blood glucose levels cause the eventual formation of advanced glycation end products (AGEs). AGEs are bonded sugar groups that stick to the proteins inside our cells. They exercise their adverse effects on our cellular metabolisms by the creation of free radicals that lead to intracellular oxidative damage. Clearly, by sacrificing the carbohydrate-laden nutrition we are so accustomed to and following more thoughtful beneficial nutritional intake, we give rise to improved or optimized health span potential.

Thus the adherence to a more beneficial discipline in any of the health optimization areas that we are focused on for our empowered well-being ultimately brings about gains. The sacrifice may appear painful at first blush because behavioral habit change is never really easy. But it is connected to the infinite law of receiving, and any suffering endured by the forfeiture will yield immeasurable benefit in the long term. Many who have followed our plan to work with their diabetes will recognize this as true. By sacrificing the overuse of carbohydrates in the nutritional intake and maintaining only the minimum necessary intake, they have routinely been able to eliminate the need for oral and injected medications that were not only considerably expensive from a financial perspective, but did not resolve the ongoing degenerative challenges caused by the elevated blood sugar levels, such as nerve damage, vascular disease, kidney failure, medication side effects, pain, depression, and so forth. We have seen numerous resolutions of adult onset diabetes by the simple discipline of a low-carbohydrate nutritional program.

Our "losses," by virtue of sacrifice, discipline, prioritization, and their ensuing behavior modifications, are replaced by immeasurably improved health outcomes and a sense of well-being that endures years beyond the perceived temporary gratification of the Twinkie sugar rush.

One of the many techniques we use to assist with this "withdrawal" is the idea of exchanging a perceived pleasure for an alternative healthy activity. Also, our use of biofeedback training modalities significantly decreases anxieties and compulsive behaviors during the transition period.

The challenges of the first weeks of the empowered medicine program are the most exhilarating. It is a time for creativity and honest introspection.

Your Empowered Medicine Cabinet

Creating Space

When we create the space for that which we desire we are sending out an intentional signal, so to speak, that we are seriously ready for this new person, experience, or thing to show up in our lives. For example, if we desire a new partner in love we would ideally shift from sleeping in the middle of the bed to sleeping on one side, thereby making room for our anticipated partner. Or, if we desire a new wardrobe, ideally we would clean out those clothes and accessories that no longer fit or no longer resonate with our sense of style.

We can take this same approach when it comes to "creating space" for our desired optimized health. Over the next several days you are going to actively participate in the law of infinite sacrifice by literally creating space for your empowered health by decluttering your space. When we set our environment up to serve us, we are able to propel ourselves even faster toward our goals. The following is a simple bulleted guide to get you started, but don't stop here. Take it even further as you are guided to do so.

Kitchen Space Clearing:

- ☐ Refrigerator—When is the last time you pulled everything out of your refrigerator, wiped down the shelves, and threw away everything that was expired, looked like a science experiment gone wrong, or you know that you know is not in alignment with your health goals? Well, now is the time to either do it for the first time, or do it again.
- ☐ Pantry—Take the same approach as you did for the refrigerator to tackle the pantry. Pull it all out, wipe it down, throw out anything that is expired. Now take it a step further and toss out white flour, white sugar, white potatoes, and white rice because no one will ever get healthy eating and baking with those. Remember, this is about you creating the space (sacrificing that which no longer serves) for that optimized, empowered health status you truly desire. So toss it—you can do it!

Wardrobe Space Clearing:

Tackle your closet! You want to make room for those new and better-fitting clothes, right? Take several hours and pull everything out of your closet. Anything that you have not worn in over a year is a definite candidate for the donation box. Now, anything you have but you do not absolutely love can also go into the donation box. Finally, anything that is too big or too small that you have been holding onto forever just in case one day … donation box.

Exception: Find one article of clothing that is in your ideal size and that you love (this could even be your bridal gown, your prom dress, your old favorite pair of jeans, or tuxedo, as the case may be). Keep this out and prominently placed so that you see it every day. Use this as your inspiration and motivation for reaching your health goals. Every time you look at this article of clothing, affirm the following, "The day I can fit into that is getting closer and closer." Or, "I am going to be rocking that outfit very soon!" Or, something comparable that resonates with you.

Clearing Other Spaces:

You can take this space clearing process to every room in your house, your office, and even your car.

CHAPTER 12

The Infinite Law of Obedience in Health

When I let go of what I am,
I become what I might be.
When I let go of what I have,
I receive what I need.

—Lao Tzu

As I approached this final chapter, I reviewed several example cases from Infinite Health Integrative Medicine Center in an effort to pick one that would be ideal here. This case, after all, should exemplify the effective use of all the universal laws. This case could or would be the foundation that springboards many of you into a more experiential application of the universal laws.

I found many cases that would exemplify different aspects of the laws and their practical implementation. But I also came across any number of additional realizations as I reviewed them. Among these I observed that many of my patients who ultimately were quite successful and seemingly more empowered in determining their desired health optimizations were those who experienced not just one but multiple setbacks or deviations over the course of their convalescence. Their determination and resolve sustained their efforts and were ultimately the key to their success. More importantly, whether it was through intuition or through their recognition of the need to implement each of the laws, the resolve and discipline these successful individuals demonstrated, and their fluency in applying theses universal laws to their personal challenges, were telling factors in the likelihood of a positive outcome.

Reaching a clear interpretation of the practical nature of each of these laws, by virtue of our own acceptance and internalization, is a key element of empowerment. This internalization facilitates implementation of directed thought and is a means of personal growth.

The personal involvement and participation with the exercises and Empowered Medicine

Cabinet activities are probably the best indicators of discipline and resolve. These processes are excellent indicators of overall success, because the individuals who succeeded with the demands of the Empowered Medicine Cabinet are the one who achieved success in health.

It always seems impossible until it's done.
—Nelson Mandela

To the mind that is still, the whole universe surrenders.
—Lao Tzu, *Tao Te Ching*

Although we are each given the template of our potential future health by our parents via their shared genomic gift, is it possible that our lives should emulate, insofar as our health is concerned, the same outcomes that our parents exhibited? We most often answer this question in the affirmative. In reality, however, this is not the case where we choose to consciously optimize the information provided to our epigenetic infrastructure that each of our cells contains.

In providing better information to our epigenetic pathways, we create improved intracellular environments, which improve the expression of our individual sets of DNA. This leads to realizing optimized health patterns, as opposed to merely accepting the genetic path of our parents and ancestors.

Barring the unfortunate dominant hereditary mishaps that do tragically occur, the development of disease resulting from epigenetic misbehavior is simply due to the laws of nature having their way with our bodies as the result of our disobedience, whether that be from a perspective of knowledge or ignorance. Our contributions to manifesting significant medical disorders, chronic or otherwise, falls uniquely on our shoulders because we quite simply have not played in a cooperative fashion using the universal laws.

If we are to benefit from the governance that has been established by a set of laws, we must be obedient to these laws. The simple understanding of the law is not in and of itself sufficient to derive benefit from it. The power of the benefit is contained in adherence to the law. The value is only acquired when that self-imposed force of submission—resolve and cost—is adequate.

It is better to conquer yourself than to win a thousand battles.
Then the victory is yours.

—Buddha

Any criminal may have knowledge of the law, but the benefit of that knowledge is reaped only by virtue of the force necessary to enact adherence—the intention to comply with the law.

This adherence enables ongoing harmony with the ideals and parameters the law establishes. In that force of adherence lies the ultimate benefit for the individual.

From a practical perspective, adherence is the ability to recognize the occasions and parameters that require obedience, and then to thoughtfully apply and enact the universal laws that have been described in the preceding chapters. If we are to activate our epigenetic infrastructures to produce the best of our genetic gifts, rather than the suboptimal ones, we must discover this thoughtful practicality in the laws. Only then will we become obedient to the law, and only then will it allow us to harmonize our pursuits of health with the health images we have created for ourselves by virtue of our inner beliefs.

In a spiritual sense, disobedience of law is considered a sin. Sins are met with the infliction of some form of punishment, the degree of which is commensurate to the degree of disobedient behavior. The punishment is the natural byproduct of the errant behavior. That is to say, when we disobey or sin, the law will dispense a compensatory penalty. That penalty would generally be in the form of illness and chronic disease or an aggravation thereof.

For example, failing to get adequate sleep results in the compromise of a number of bodily functions. Epigenetic alterations from lack of sleep lead to metabolic, inflammatory, immune, and stress-related compromise in our bodies. These epigenetic alterations may be the cause of the cardiovascular disease, obesity, and cognitive decline seen in people who are sleep deprived.

Disobedience of different laws result in different penalties. The torment endured by each "sin" may be of assistance in the interpretation of the law that has been disobeyed. And practically speaking, we can more readily recognize our failures after the fact. Do not despair! Our failures are the best professors we have and readily lead us to success. For example, disobedience of the law of allowance will likely lead to aggravations of many ongoing chronic medical problems. Fighting (resisting) the problem—such as diabetes—will create a stress response, and as previously discussed, elevate cortisol, adrenaline, and growth hormone to degrees that will impede the activity of endogenous insulin and aggravate the blood sugar levels.

The more resistant we are to our challenges, the more stress responses we will endure. This is precisely driven by the law of allowance, and our disobedience thereof.

In order to achieve consistent health we need only be sufficiently intent on attracting that health we desire. Doing so is obedient to the law of attraction and the law of supply. Desire, intent, and expectation are the driving components of these laws. The imaging exercises suggested in this book assist in maintenance of focus and intent on the desired outcomes.

Desire and expect awesome health, particularly in the imaging exercises. Worry, a lack mentality, affirming adverse outcomes, and doubting an optimized health outcome are all blocks and limitations to acquiring dynamic, empowered health. Doubt in particular impedes and stifles desired health. For this reason, we must maintain entourages of supportive individuals who reinforce our beliefs and goals.

This is particularly true for those of us with multiple problems for which our physician(s) give us nihilistic prognoses. We must believe before we see (law of supply), and I am the first to admit that physicians are all too happy to focus on the negative as we discussed before. This setting, of course, requires us to work with those physicians who are willing to support and empower our desires and expectations, as well as the statistical data.

In a setting in which our thoughts are filled with the perception of chaotic health outcomes—ones that are continuously detrimental and adverse in nature—we are not abiding by the law of thinking, particularly in the sense that our thinking is not uniformly picturing our idealized health images (law of supply). Understanding and obeying this law formalizes our abilities to proactively create empowered, optimized health from the creative affirmative images we have in our minds. Disobedience of these two laws creates the perception of randomness in our health outcomes. We then become subject to all manner of diversity in illness that may be imagined. I generally compare this to being at sea in a rudderless skiff that has no means of propulsion and is just waiting for the next wave to wash over it.

Conveniently, any adverse outcomes may also be easily traced, after the fact, to the disobedient mind-set. This "tracking" ability enables us to forgive and correct the nefarious mind-set, easily bringing about the understanding that we are never victims of randomness where our states of health are concerned.

When we have delays in acquiring the health outcomes we desire or in obtaining alternative results from those imagined, this generally reflects a failure to obey the law of compensation. Look to the methods employed as the causative origin of failure in this case, as the corrective modalities chosen may actually lead to even better outcomes than originally anticipated.

Knowledge of these laws enables us to find pathways of failure, and more important, perspective on improvements that we may use to acquire the optimized road to recovery and convalescence. Most of these paths are unseen at the time of, or before, our failures or successes.

These laws are at work for every decision, thought, and action we may take, whether we are conscious of it or not. Knowing and obeying them is to our collective benefit, giving us the edge over happenstance and hazard. By their habitual use, we take charge of the elements of success in our lives and thus become creators of our health and not simply the coconspirators of perceived randomness. Ultimately, this guidance empowers us all to take charge of our health and well-being in a manner that assures success.

The thought (law of thinking) and expectation (law of supply and law of attraction) of extraordinary health and well-being gives rise to just that with adherence (law of receiving and law of increase) to the image created. Ultimately, the health we obtain (law of compensation) in the setting of this newfound obedient behavior (law of forgiveness) will replace the issues created (law of sacrifice) by our historically disobedient behaviors. And by consistent application of the laws, our new behaviors allow (law of allowance) the laws to work to our benefit.

APPENDIX

Fourteen-Day Gratitude Journal

Day 1

> *Whoever has gratitude for their health and their body will be given more, and will have an abundance of health to their body.*
> —Rhonda Byrne, author of *The Magic*

1. I am so thankful and grateful for:_____

   _____,

   because_____

   _____.

   Thank you, thank you, thank you.

2. I am so thankful and grateful for:_____

   _____,

   because_____

   _____.

   Thank you, thank you, thank you.

3. I am so thankful and grateful for:_____

   _____,

   because_____

   _____.

   Thank you, thank you, thank you.

4. I am so thankful and grateful for:_____

   _____,

   because_____

   _____.

   Thank you, thank you, thank you.

5. I am so thankful and grateful for:_____
   _____,

   because_____
   _____.

   Thank you, thank you, thank you.

6. I am so thankful and grateful for:_____
   _____,

   because_____
   _____.

   Thank you, thank you, thank you.

7. I am so thankful and grateful for:_____
   _____,

   because_____
   _____.

   Thank you, thank you, thank you.

8. I am so thankful and grateful for:_____
   _____,

   because_____
   _____.

   Thank you, thank you, thank you.

9. I am so thankful and grateful for:_____
   _____,

   because_____
   _____.

   Thank you, thank you, thank you.

10. I am so thankful and grateful for:_____
    _____,

    because_____
    _____.

    Thank you, thank you, thank you.

Day 2

Natural forces within us are the true healers.

—Hippocrates

1. I am so thankful and grateful for:_____

   _____

   because_____

   _____.

   Thank you, thank you, thank you.

2. I am so thankful and grateful for:_____

   _____

   because_____

   _____.

   Thank you, thank you, thank you.

3. I am so thankful and grateful for:_____

   _____

   because_____

   _____.

   Thank you, thank you, thank you.

4. I am so thankful and grateful for:_____

   _____

   because_____

   _____.

   Thank you, thank you, thank you.

5. I am so thankful and grateful for:_____

   _____

   because_____

   _____.

   Thank you, thank you, thank you.

6. I am so thankful and grateful for:_____
_____
because_____
_____.

Thank you, thank you, thank you.

7. I am so thankful and grateful for:_____
_____
because_____
_____.

Thank you, thank you, thank you.

8. I am so thankful and grateful for:_____
_____
because_____
_____.

Thank you, thank you, thank you.

9. I am so thankful and grateful for:_____
_____
because_____
_____.

Thank you, thank you, thank you.

10. I am so thankful and grateful for:_____
_____
because_____
_____.

Thank you, thank you, thank you.

Day 3

The world is full of magical things waiting for our wits to grow sharper.
—Eden Phillpotts

1. I am so thankful and grateful for:_____

    _____

    because_____

    _____.

    Thank you, thank you, thank you.

2. I am so thankful and grateful for:_____

    _____

    because_____

    _____.

    Thank you, thank you, thank you.

3. I am so thankful and grateful for:_____

    _____

    because_____

    _____.

    Thank you, thank you, thank you.

4. I am so thankful and grateful for:_____

    _____

    because_____

    _____.

    Thank you, thank you, thank you.

5. I am so thankful and grateful for:_____

    _____

    because_____

    _____.

    Thank you, thank you, thank you.

6. I am so thankful and grateful for:_____

_____

because_____

_____.

Thank you, thank you, thank you.

7. I am so thankful and grateful for:_____

_____

because_____

_____.

Thank you, thank you, thank you.

8. I am so thankful and grateful for:_____

_____

because_____

_____.

Thank you, thank you, thank you.

9. I am so thankful and grateful for:_____

_____

because_____

_____.

Thank you, thank you, thank you.

10. I am so thankful and grateful for:_____

_____

because_____

_____.

Thank you, thank you, thank you.

Day 4

A hundred times every day I remind myself that my inner and outer life depends
on the labors of other men, living and dead, and that I must exert myself in order
to give the same measure as I have received and
am still receiving.

—Albert Einstein

1. I am so thankful and grateful for:_____

    _____

    because_____

    _____.

    Thank you, thank you, thank you.

2. I am so thankful and grateful for:_____

    _____

    because_____

    _____.

    Thank you, thank you, thank you.

3. I am so thankful and grateful for:_____

    _____

    because_____

    _____.

    Thank you, thank you, thank you.

4. I am so thankful and grateful for:_____

    _____

    because_____

    _____.

    Thank you, thank you, thank you.

5. I am so thankful and grateful for:_____

    _____

    because_____

    _____.

    Thank you, thank you, thank you.

6. I am so thankful and grateful for:_____

_____

because_____

_____.

Thank you, thank you, thank you.

7. I am so thankful and grateful for:_____

_____

because_____

_____.

Thank you, thank you, thank you.

8. I am so thankful and grateful for:_____

_____

because_____

_____.

Thank you, thank you, thank you.

9. I am so thankful and grateful for:_____

_____

because_____

_____.

Thank you, thank you, thank you.

10. I am so thankful and grateful for:_____

_____

because_____

_____.

Thank you, thank you, thank you.

Day 5

God gave you a gift of 86,400 seconds today.
Have you used one to say "thank you"?

—William Ward

1. I am so thankful and grateful for:_____

_____

because_____

_____.

Thank you, thank you, thank you.

2. I am so thankful and grateful for:_____

_____

because_____

_____.

Thank you, thank you, thank you.

3. I am so thankful and grateful for:_____

_____

because_____

_____.

Thank you, thank you, thank you.

4. I am so thankful and grateful for:_____

_____

because_____

_____.

Thank you, thank you, thank you.

5. I am so thankful and grateful for:_____

_____

because_____

_____.

Thank you, thank you, thank you.

6. I am so thankful and grateful for:_____

   _____

   because_____

   _____.

   Thank you, thank you, thank you.

7. I am so thankful and grateful for:_____

   _____

   because_____

   _____.

   Thank you, thank you, thank you.

8. I am so thankful and grateful for:_____

   _____

   because_____

   _____.

   Thank you, thank you, thank you.

9. I am so thankful and grateful for:_____

   _____

   because_____

   _____.

   Thank you, thank you, thank you.

10. I am so thankful and grateful for:_____

    _____

    because_____

    _____.

    Thank you, thank you, thank you.

Day 6

Gratitude is the memory of the heart.
—Jean-Baptiste Massieu

1. I am so thankful and grateful for:_____

   _____

   because_____

   _____.

   Thank you, thank you, thank you.

2. I am so thankful and grateful for:_____

   _____

   because_____

   _____.

   Thank you, thank you, thank you.

3. I am so thankful and grateful for:_____

   _____

   because_____

   _____.

   Thank you, thank you, thank you.

4. I am so thankful and grateful for:_____

   _____

   because_____

   _____.

   Thank you, thank you, thank you.

5. I am so thankful and grateful for:_____

   _____

   because_____

   _____.

   Thank you, thank you, thank you.

6. I am so thankful and grateful for:_____

_____

because_____

_____.

Thank you, thank you, thank you.

7. I am so thankful and grateful for:_____

_____

because_____

_____.

Thank you, thank you, thank you.

8. I am so thankful and grateful for:_____

_____

because_____

_____.

Thank you, thank you, thank you.

9. I am so thankful and grateful for:_____

_____

because_____

_____.

Thank you, thank you, thank you.

10. I am so thankful and grateful for:_____

_____

because_____

_____.

Thank you, thank you, thank you.

Day 7

You say grace before meals. All right. But I say grace before the concert and the opera, and grace before the play and pantomime, and grace before I open a book, and grace before sketching, painting, swimming, fencing, boxing, walking, playing, dancing, and grace before I dip the pen in the ink.

—G. K. Chesterson

1. I am so thankful and grateful for:_____

   _____

   because_____

   _____.

   Thank you, thank you, thank you.

2. I am so thankful and grateful for:_____

   _____

   because_____

   _____.

   Thank you, thank you, thank you.

3. I am so thankful and grateful for:_____

   _____

   because_____

   _____.

   Thank you, thank you, thank you.

4. I am so thankful and grateful for:_____

   _____

   because_____

   _____.

   Thank you, thank you, thank you.

5. I am so thankful and grateful for:_____

   _____

   because_____

   _____.

   Thank you, thank you, thank you.

6. I am so thankful and grateful for:_____
_____

because_____
_____.

Thank you, thank you, thank you.

7. I am so thankful and grateful for:_____
_____

because_____
_____.

Thank you, thank you, thank you.

8. I am so thankful and grateful for:_____
_____

because_____
_____.

Thank you, thank you, thank you.

9. I am so thankful and grateful for:_____
_____

because_____
_____.

Thank you, thank you, thank you.

10. I am so thankful and grateful for:_____
_____

because_____
_____.

Thank you, thank you, thank you.

Day 8

People who wait for a magic wand fail to see that they are the magic wand.
—Thomas Leonard

1. I am so thankful and grateful for:_____

    _____

    because_____

    _____.

    Thank you, thank you, thank you.

2. I am so thankful and grateful for:_____

    _____

    because_____

    _____.

    Thank you, thank you, thank you.

3. I am so thankful and grateful for:_____

    _____

    because_____

    _____.

    Thank you, thank you, thank you.

4. I am so thankful and grateful for:_____

    _____

    because_____

    _____.

    Thank you, thank you, thank you.

5. I am so thankful and grateful for:_____

    _____

    because_____

    _____.

    Thank you, thank you, thank you.

6. I am so thankful and grateful for:_____

_____

because_____

_____.

Thank you, thank you, thank you.

7. I am so thankful and grateful for:_____

_____

because_____

_____.

Thank you, thank you, thank you.

8. I am so thankful and grateful for:_____

_____

because_____

_____.

Thank you, thank you, thank you.

9. I am so thankful and grateful for:_____

_____

because_____

_____.

Thank you, thank you, thank you.

10. I am so thankful and grateful for:_____

_____

because_____

_____.

Thank you, thank you, thank you.

Day 9

Turn your wounds into wisdom.

—Oprah Winfrey

1. I am so thankful and grateful for:_____

   _____

   because_____

   _____.

   Thank you, thank you, thank you.

2. I am so thankful and grateful for:_____

   _____

   because_____

   _____.

   Thank you, thank you, thank you.

3. I am so thankful and grateful for:_____

   _____

   because_____

   _____.

   Thank you, thank you, thank you.

4. I am so thankful and grateful for:_____

   _____

   because_____

   _____.

   Thank you, thank you, thank you.

5. I am so thankful and grateful for:_____

   _____

   because_____

   _____.

   Thank you, thank you, thank you.

6. I am so thankful and grateful for:_____
_____
because_____
_____.
Thank you, thank you, thank you.

7. I am so thankful and grateful for:_____
_____
because_____
_____.
Thank you, thank you, thank you.

8. I am so thankful and grateful for:_____
_____
because_____
_____.
Thank you, thank you, thank you.

9. I am so thankful and grateful for:_____
_____
because_____
_____.
Thank you, thank you, thank you.

10. I am so thankful and grateful for:_____
_____
because_____
_____.
Thank you, thank you, thank you.

Day 10

To speak gratitude is courteous and pleasant, to enact gratitude is generous and noble, but to live gratitude is to touch Heaven.

—Johannes A. Gaertner

1. I am so thankful and grateful for:_____

   _____

   because_____

   _____.

   Thank you, thank you, thank you.

2. I am so thankful and grateful for:_____

   _____

   because_____

   _____.

   Thank you, thank you, thank you.

3. I am so thankful and grateful for:_____

   _____

   because_____

   _____.

   Thank you, thank you, thank you.

4. I am so thankful and grateful for:_____

   _____

   because_____

   _____.

   Thank you, thank you, thank you.

5. I am so thankful and grateful for:_____

   _____

   because_____

   _____.

   Thank you, thank you, thank you.

6. I am so thankful and grateful for:_____

_____

because_____

_____.

Thank you, thank you, thank you.

7. I am so thankful and grateful for:_____

_____

because_____

_____.

Thank you, thank you, thank you.

8. I am so thankful and grateful for:_____

_____

because_____

_____.

Thank you, thank you, thank you.

9. I am so thankful and grateful for:_____

_____

because_____

_____.

Thank you, thank you, thank you.

10. I am so thankful and grateful for:_____

_____

because_____

_____.

Thank you, thank you, thank you.

Day 11

We showed him (i.e. man) the way:
whether he be grateful or ungrateful (rests on his will).

—Unknown

1. I am so thankful and grateful for:_____

   _____

   because_____

   _____.

   Thank you, thank you, thank you.

2. I am so thankful and grateful for:_____

   _____

   because_____

   _____.

   Thank you, thank you, thank you.

3. I am so thankful and grateful for:_____

   _____

   because_____

   _____.

   Thank you, thank you, thank you.

4. I am so thankful and grateful for:_____

   _____

   because_____

   _____.

   Thank you, thank you, thank you.

5. I am so thankful and grateful for:_____

   _____

   because_____

   _____.

   Thank you, thank you, thank you.

6. I am so thankful and grateful for:_____
_____
because_____
_____.

Thank you, thank you, thank you.

7. I am so thankful and grateful for:_____
_____
because_____
_____.

Thank you, thank you, thank you.

8. I am so thankful and grateful for:_____
_____
because_____
_____.

Thank you, thank you, thank you.

9. I am so thankful and grateful for:_____
_____
because_____
_____.

Thank you, thank you, thank you.

10. I am so thankful and grateful for:_____
_____
because_____
_____.

Thank you, thank you, thank you.

Day 12

When you arise in the morning, give thanks for the morning light, for your life and strength. Give thanks for your food and the joy of living. If you see no reason for giving thanks, the fault lies within yourself.

—Tecumseh

1. I am so thankful and grateful for:_____
   _____
   because_____
   _____.
   Thank you, thank you, thank you.

2. I am so thankful and grateful for:_____
   _____
   because_____
   _____.
   Thank you, thank you, thank you.

3. I am so thankful and grateful for:_____
   _____
   because_____
   _____.
   Thank you, thank you, thank you.

4. I am so thankful and grateful for:_____
   _____
   because_____
   _____.
   Thank you, thank you, thank you.

5. I am so thankful and grateful for:_____
   _____
   because_____
   _____.
   Thank you, thank you, thank you.

6. I am so thankful and grateful for:_____
_____
because_____
_____.
Thank you, thank you, thank you.

7. I am so thankful and grateful for:_____
_____
because_____
_____.
Thank you, thank you, thank you.

8. I am so thankful and grateful for:_____
_____
because_____
_____.
Thank you, thank you, thank you.

9. I am so thankful and grateful for:_____
_____
because_____
_____.
Thank you, thank you, thank you.

10. I am so thankful and grateful for:_____
_____
because_____
_____.
Thank you, thank you, thank you.

Day 13

1. I am so thankful and grateful for:_____

    _____

    because_____

    _____.

    Thank you, thank you, thank you.

2. I am so thankful and grateful for:_____

    _____

    because_____

    _____.

    Thank you, thank you, thank you.

3. I am so thankful and grateful for:_____

    _____

    because_____

    _____.

    Thank you, thank you, thank you.

4. I am so thankful and grateful for:_____

    _____

    because_____

    _____.

    Thank you, thank you, thank you.

5. I am so thankful and grateful for:_____

    _____

    because_____

    _____.

    Thank you, thank you, thank you.

6. I am so thankful and grateful for:_____

    _____

    because_____

    _____.

    Thank you, thank you, thank you.

7. I am so thankful and grateful for:_____

    _____

    because_____

    _____.

    Thank you, thank you, thank you.

8. I am so thankful and grateful for:_____

    _____

    because_____

    _____.

    Thank you, thank you, thank you.

9. I am so thankful and grateful for:_____

    _____

    because_____

    _____.

    Thank you, thank you, thank you.

10. I am so thankful and grateful for:_____

    _____

    because_____

    _____.

    Thank you, thank you, thank you.

Day 14

When I started counting my blessings, my whole life turned around.

—Willie Nelson

1. I am so thankful and grateful for:_____
   _____
   because_____
   _____.
   Thank you, thank you, thank you.

2. I am so thankful and grateful for:_____
   _____
   because_____
   _____.
   Thank you, thank you, thank you.

3. I am so thankful and grateful for:_____
   _____
   because_____
   _____.
   Thank you, thank you, thank you.

4. I am so thankful and grateful for:_____
   _____
   because_____
   _____.
   Thank you, thank you, thank you.

5. I am so thankful and grateful for:_____
   _____
   because_____
   _____.
   Thank you, thank you, thank you.

6. I am so thankful and grateful for:_____
   _____
   because_____
   _____.
   Thank you, thank you, thank you.

7. I am so thankful and grateful for:_____
   _____
   because_____
   _____.
   Thank you, thank you, thank you.

8. I am so thankful and grateful for:_____
   _____
   because_____
   _____.
   Thank you, thank you, thank you.

9. I am so thankful and grateful for:_____
   _____
   because_____
   _____.
   Thank you, thank you, thank you.

10. I am so thankful and grateful for:_____
    _____
    because_____
    _____.
    Thank you, thank you, thank you.

Congratulations! You have completed the Fourteen-Day Empowered Medicine Gratitude Journal! But don't stop here! Keep it up every day and watch more and more infinite health begin to flow to you!

REFERENCES

Beecher H. K. The Powerful Placebo. *JAMA*. 1955:159(17):1602–1606. doi:10.1001/jama.1955.02960340022006

Braden, Gregg, *The Spontaneous Healing of Belief,* Hay House, 2008.

Canfield, Jack, *The Success Principles,*

Chopra, Deepak, *The Seven Spiritual Laws of Success*, Amber-Allen Publishing and New World Library, 1994.

Cohen S., Janicki-Deverts D., Miller, G. E., "Psychological Stress and Disease." *JAMA*.2007:298(14):1685–1687. doi:10.1001/jama.298.14.1685.

DeMaria, Eric J. MD; Sugerman, Harvey J. MD; Meador, Jill G. RN, BSN; Doty, James M. MD; Kellum, John M. MD; Wolfe, Luke MS; Szucs, Richard A. MD; Turner, Mary Ann MD. "High Failure Rate After Laparoscopic Adjustable Silicone Gastric Banding for Treatment of Morbid Obesity." *Annals of Surgery*: June 2001 Vol. 233 - Issue 6 - pp 809–818

The emperor's new drugs: An analysis of antidepressant medication data submitted to the U.S. Food and Drug Administration.

http://www.emersoncentral.com/compensation.htm

http://www.emersoncentral.com/spirituallaws.htm

http://www.goodreads.com/quotes/201777-i-ve-had-a-lot-of-worries-in-my-life-most

http://www.goodreads.com/quotes/374489-the-greatest-revolution-of-our-generation-is-the-discovery-that

http://science.sciencemag.org/content/291/5507/1304.full

Kirsch, Irving; Moore, Thomas J.; Scoboria, Alan; Nicholls, Sarah S. *Prevention & Treatment*, Vol 5(1), Jul 2002, No Pagination Specified Article 23. http://dx.doi.org/10.1037/1522–3736.5.1.523a

Medawar, P., *The Limits of Science* pg 98 (New York Harper and Row) 1984 Taken from Wiki quote at https://en.wikiquote.org/wiki/Peter_Medawar

Miller, F. G., "William James, Faith, and the Placebo Effect," *Perspectives in Biology and Medicine*, Vol. 48 no. 2 Spring 2005, pp 273–281.

Möller-Levet, Carla S., Archer, Simon N., Bucca, Giselda, Laing, Emma E., Slak, Ana, Kabiljo, Renata, Lo, June C. Y., Santhi, Nayantara, von Schantz, Malcolm, Smith, Colin P., and Dijk, Derk-Jan. "Effects of insufficient sleep on circadian rhythmicity and expression amplitude of the human blood transcriptome." PNAS 2013 110 (12) E1132-E1141; published ahead of print February 25, 2013,doi:10.1073/pnas.1217154110

Nerurkar A, Bitton A, Davis RB, Phillips RS, Yeh G. "When Physicians Counsel About Stress: Results of a National Study." *JAMA Intern Med.* 2013;173(1):76–77. doi:10.1001/2013.jamainternmed.480

Suter, M., Calmes, J.M., Paroz, A. et. al. "A 10-year Experience with Laparoscopic Gastric Banding for Morbid Obesity: High Long-Term Complication and Failure Rates." OBES SURG (2006) 16: 829. doi:10.1381/096089206777822359

Printed in the United States
By Bookmasters